A Bitter Harvest:
Pesticides & Cancer – Avoidable Human Suffering
by
Ron Wooten-Green, Ph.D.

A Bitter Harvest at Troublesome Creek

Table of Contents

Dedication & Caveat # 1

Dedication:

This book is dedicated to the people cited within these pages:

- Donna Jo * Shelley   * Susan   * Duane
- JoAn   * Sandra   * Helen & Ben

And the millions of others who, through no fault of their own, have suffered and died needlessly.

Caveat #1:

As will become clear, this book comes with a certain point of view, a slant evident in the dedication above. It is a perspective, this writer believes, shared by most, if not all, who have devoted much of their lives caring for the terminally ill – especially those dying of cancer. An open admission is hereby served: this book is a subjective presentation of a critical public health issue; yet grounded in objective facts. Total objectivity has been eroded by the reality of approximately 1000 bedside experiences.

As Pete Seeger noted nearly 60 years ago in a lecture at Teachers College, Columbia University:

There is no such thing as pure objectivity,
and there are two sides to every question.
Of course, in my opinion,
there are two sides to a piece of flypaper too,
and it makes a great difference to the fly which side he lands on.[1]

---

[1] Pete Seeger, "The Columbia Concert, 1961" Pete Seeger: In His Own Words, Selected and Edited by Rob Rosenthal and Sam Rosenthal, Boulder, CO: Paradigm Publishers, 2012), 251.

Introduction

The inspiration for this book unfolded gradually while the author was working as a hospice chaplain in a nine-county area of Southwest Iowa and Northeast Nebraska. At one point, our staff realized that we were dealing with an unusual number of young women dying of cancer of the reproductive organs. We wondered: "Is this a cancer pocket?"

As a chaplain, I had the privilege to work very closely with these young women and their families. It was a relationship based on trust and a willingness to listen to the cares, concerns, fears, and the pain of dashed dreams. There were those who were trying to make sense out of the senseless: "What did I do wrong?" "Why is this happening to Mom?" "Why is God doing this to my wife?" "Is there something in the air? Something in the water?" Others were quite clear on the matter: "It's the chemicals," they said.

Research was called for, and so it began. The families of the now deceased young women were given the opportunity to vent and to speculate. In addition, extensive research into the history and dynamics of cancer, the history of chemical use on the croplands of America, the governmental regulation of pesticides, medical and scientific research and related issues, such as politics, was conducted. Anecdotal material gathered from the patients and families reveal the depth of the human tragedies. The stories found herein are representative of the millions of people in similar situations.

Caveat # 2:

While this book cannot address all forms of cancer and their causes in-depth, no more than it can examine each of the thousands of chemicals and their relationships to human health, it can draw attention to how certain political and corporate forces, policies and practices, significantly contribute to an increasingly pernicious environment world-wide. While we deal here somewhat tangentially with the medical sciences, biological research, and agricultural practices, the primary focus and concern is with the costs to humanity.

In the end, this book provides a "way through" the morass and utter mess we have made of our farms, lawns, gardens, environment and economy with our dedication to the myth that happiness, prosperity, and well-being can be obtained through chemistry. Finally, an accounting is called for, politically, economically and socially. We must stop what we are doing. When calculating the costs of doing agribusiness, we must include the human costs of chemicals affecting public health. By throwing more and more chemicals at the problems of pests and growing food, we approach a definition of insanity often attributed to Albert Einstein:

Doing the same thing over-and-over again,
and expecting different results.

By the same token, we must especially stop what we are NOT doing. Yogi Berra, great baseball catcher that he was, became, perhaps, even better known for his verbal head-spinning philosophical pitches as manager of the often-hapless NY Mets. When asked by a reporter how he felt about the fact that hardly any fans were turning out to watch his faltering team losing game-after-game, Yogi replied: "If people don't want to come out to the ballpark, how are you going to stop them?"[2]

The same question may be raised here: If people don't want to stop what they are not doing, how are we going to stop them? This book offers alternatives for ending the insanity of our ways.

---

[2] Baseball Almanac: www:baseball-almanac.com/quotes/quoberra.

Tables

Chapter One

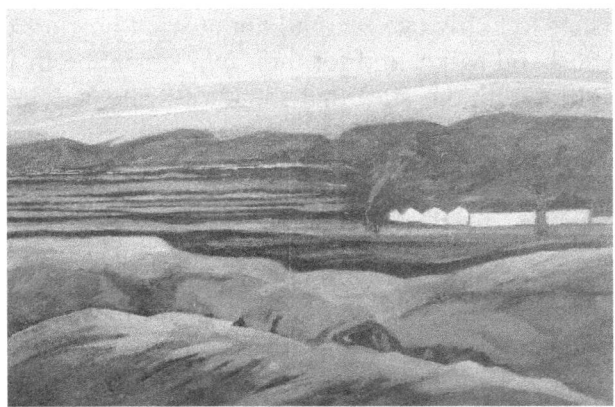

Harvest,

Stories of Hope & Hopelessness:
Promises, Pesticides, Pollution, and Pain

Everybody knows that the dice are loaded
Everybody knows that the Plague is coming.
Everybody knows that it is moving fast…
Everybody knows that you're in trouble…
Everybody knows that it's coming apart….[3]

The mystery began to unfold as this writer worked as a hospice chaplain covering nine counties in southwest Iowa, and another six in eastern Nebraska. She arrived in a wheel chair at our hospice office in Council Bluffs, Iowa. Little did we know, at the time, that the immobilized woman in that chair was to be the first of many of her neighbors seeking end-of-life care. We thought this 56-year-old woman was far too young to be losing her battle against cancer. Little did we know! In the days and weeks ahead, we were to meet and provide care for women far younger than Donna Jo, but virtual neighbors of one another.

DONNA JO (1940-1998)

---

[3] Leonard Cohen, "Everybody Knows," Leonard Cohen: I'm Your Man (CBS Records, [now Sony], 1988); booklet, p.4.

September 1997: She insists on going to hospice rather than having hospice come to her. She wants to meet the entire staff on their own turf. She wishes to know every detail about what hospice can do for her, for her husband Mike, and for their two sons. She insists on making the point with our staff that she knows she is dying. But she also wants us to know that she is not about to roll over and die, that she still has a lot of living to do; and she has come to us wanting help to do that living in the very best way possible.

Donna Jo presents herself with the demeanor of a woman very much in the habit of being in control of her life; of knowing what she will and will not do; of clarifying with those around her what she wants and does not want. It is certain within a very few minutes that she desires to be in control of her dying. From this point on it is a rare thing for any staff member to refer to Donna Jo as a "patient." The term, somehow, just doesn't fit.

Mike explains that Donna Jo is a successful journalist and a talented vocalist. They had met at Sidney High School only a few miles from where they now live in Fremont county, Iowa. They had lived on the East coast for many years while Mike was practicing law. Shortly after moving his law practice to Kansas City, Donna Jo was diagnosed with ovarian cancer. She was 55 years old. Looking back, first symptoms appeared when she was 40.

There appears to be only one issue that is troubling Donna Jo. She has no idea where the cancer came from. There is no history of it in her family. "I keep wondering: What did I do wrong?"

After checking us all out very carefully, Donna Jo apparently decides we are an OK bunch, and asks, "Where do I sign up?" Later, as Mike is wheeling her toward the front door, she turns to me and asks, "Could you come to see me day after tomorrow?"

She looks so very vital and alive, a beautiful brunette with a broad smile and a twinkling in her eyes that light up the room. With Mike and the boys gathered around her, there is the sense that this mother and wife has the world by the tail.

Life is very different now. I am viewing that which **was** – a 1985 oil painting of Donna Jo and her family. The painting is huge. It takes up almost the entire wall at the side of her hospital bed in the living room in a home where, indeed, Donna Jo had done a great deal of living. This is the farm home of her childhood, where her mother nurtured Donna Jo into a self-confident and capable young woman. The living room is different now. It is Donna Jo's dying room.

She is frail of body, in fact a skeletal version of the Donna Jo in the painting, but she is still very strong of mind and spirit. She is preparing in the best way she knows how, to ride off into the sunset of life in the style of the Rodeo Queen of her youth. She wants to "do it right," she says. She is getting ready to "saddle up" for her Last Ride. Donna Jo is ready to go.

As we talk and as we pray before I leave, I have heard some of her story – a story of much hope and promise, accomplishment and satisfaction, dreams and now shattered dreams. I have also heard the all-too-familiar companion questions: "Why has this happened to me? What did I do wrong." These are the questions raised by victims, unintentionally setting themselves up for one more victimization, the judgment that they are somehow responsible for the cancer that is ravishing their bodies.

Two years after she died, I called Mike to ask if he would be willing to fill me in on more of the details of Donna Jo's life. In the intervening years our hospice cared for several women in the same geographic area; all 15-20 years younger than Donna Jo and dying of cancer of the reproductive organs. I too wanted to know why.

Upon arriving, I am struck by the familiarity of the house and terrain. The white-sided ranch-style home with redwood stairs leading up to the front door and its surrounding yard appears to be even more immaculate and meticulously cared for than I remembered from my many visits. The interior of the home has received similar care. The painting, however, no longer adorns the wall of the living room; perhaps the memories are yet too raw.

As Mike shares Donna Jo's story, the following picture comes into focus:

June 21, 1940: Marian has just finished spraying the cows' bellies with the wonderfully effective new chemical, DDT, to keep the flies from annoying the animals, and the cows, in turn, imperiling herself and her husband, Don, with unexpected kicks that could spill both the milk and the milker. "What did we ever do without this stuff," she idly asks Don. "It is so simple & safe. Have you noticed? No bugs, no flies in the house? That is, as long as I keep it sprayed!"

It was only three years earlier in 1938 that Swiss chemist Paul Muller had introduced DDT to the world, the miracle chemical. Don and Marian were only two of millions of people who came to appreciate this chemical's power to simplify life. From its creation in 1938 through 1972, 4/4 billion pounds of DDT were added to the once pristine American landscape.[4] Despite the fact that as early as 1951, when Donna Jo was 10 years old, DDT had been discovered in alarming rates in human breast milk[5]; and despite the even more alarming warning issued in 1964 by two scientists, W.C. Hueper and W.D. Conway, that:

Cancers of all types and all causes display ... all the characteristics of an epidemic in slow motion...(fueled by) increasing contamination of the human environment with chemical and physical carcinogens....[6]

As she herds the cows down the hill to the back pasture, Marian is struck by the beauty of the deep green colors of the nearly knee-high growth of corn surrounding her view. Then, she is stricken by something far less pleasing. At first, she thinks it is a reaction to inhaling the DDT spray; sometimes it makes her feel a bit nauseous. Sickness to the stomach is an all-too-familiar feeling for her these days. After all, she is nearly 8 months pregnant with their first and, as the twists and turns of fate will have it, their last and only child.

This pain is different. It couldn't be worse than if one of the cows had kicked her in the stomach. Suddenly, Marian is in the dirt, screaming in pain and panic. "This can't be happening," she protests, "my baby's not due for another four weeks!"

But, it is happening! By the time Don reaches her side, Marian is well into labor. Managing to carry her home and placing

---

[4] Lewis G. Regenstein, <u>Cleaning Up America</u> (NY: Acropolis Books, 1993), 338.
[5] E.P Laug, et all, "Occurrence of DDT in Human Fat and Milk," <u>A.M.A. Archives of Industrial Hygiene and Occupational Medicine</u> 3 (1951), 245-46.
[6] W.C. Hueper and W.D. Conway, <u>Chemical Carcinogenesis and Cancers</u> (NY: Charles Thomas, 1964), 17, 158.

her in bed, Don then calls the doctor. Soon after his arrival, from Shenandoah (a ten-mile journey), Donna Jo makes hers.

These were happy times – a time when Marian, Don and Donna Jo were making a life for themselves. It may be imagined that happiness seemed to sprout and grow, as did the thriving garden to the west side of the farmhouse. The future seemed as limitless as their backyard view of the Nishnabotna Valley.

Perhaps, Marian and Don should have seen it coming that very September 1939 evening when they made love, almost knowing beyond doubt that a child would be conceived. However, prior to going to bed, Don turned on the radio to listen to the evening news.

He is listening to Walter Winchell's trademark greeting and is immediately chilled by Winchell's tone: "Good evening, Mr. & Mrs. America, from border to border and coast to coast, and all the ships at sea. Let's go to press!" Marian & Don learn that Germany has massed troops on the Polish border and there is, according to Winchell, a chance this could lead to another global conflict, possibly World War II.

So it was that Donna Jo had been conceived on the day some consider the real beginning of the Second World War in the space of 30+ years. Before Donna Jo turned 18 months old, Japanese planes struck at Pearl Harbor and her father enlisted in the US Navy. When she was almost two years-old, she and her mother attended Don's commissioning ceremony, as he shipped out. Don kissed them goodbye. It was the last they were ever to see him. Don's ship was sunk in the Pacific by a Japanese torpedo.

Donna Jo was a precocious child – inquisitive, adventurous, full of life and enjoying every minute of it. At a very early age she demonstrated an astounding gift for memorizing poetry and lyrics to songs; her voice often carried across the rolling Iowa farmland, competing with the skylarks, jays, and crows for center stage in their mutual daily songfests.

Mike recalled Donna Jo's stories of how she loved playing in the fields, except on those days when the crop duster saturated the land with foul-smelling chemicals scaring-off her friends, the birds. The mist from the spray was irritating to her eyes and throat. She had often wondered if the mist might be responsible for the occasional dead bird she found in the fields, along the side of the road, in the yard; or had the roar of the planes scared her winged friends to death?

It is with deep regret that Mike now recalls it was his father who flew the crop duster. Worse yet, Mike helped his father load the chemicals onto the plane. Indeed, he had often flown with his father over this very farm.

As she stood at the well in the backyard, bringing up a bucket of clear cold water on late summer day in 1945, Donna Jo looked across the valley spread out before her. She wondered what life was going to be like in that square building off to the west on the bottomland. She was eager to begin going to the Prairie Township School cozily enveloped by the ever-familiar cornfields.

While she was fascinated with what the future might hold for her in that one-room schoolhouse, she feared it as well. But at least there was a neat water well down there with equally fresh clear cold water.

She did not, of course know that, as of the 1946-47 school year, American women were already running three times the risk of having breast cancer than was true for their great-grandmothers.[7] Nor could she have known that, beginning the year of her residency in her mother's womb, breast cancer deaths were already increasing one percent yearly and would continue doing so into the 1990's.[8]

For the next six years, Donna Jo traveled the short distance from home to school, excelling in everything she touched. But one summer day in 1949 she noticed, while standing next to the well at home, that the luxurious grape arbor running southwest of the well was looking ill. The leaves had taken on a sickly mottled discoloration. She had never seen the vines look this way. Neither had Marian. They would never see the vines again. The best the County Agent could figure out, the grape arbor on this farm had become victim to neighboring farmers' use of 2-4D, a DDT-based pesticide. Never mind that Marian had never used it on her farm; financially, she could not afford it.

By the fall of 1953, Donna Jo had graduated from the little bottomland school. Traveling over the hill to the west, she entered

---

[7] Sandra Steingraber, Living Downstream: A Scientist's Personal Investigation of Cancer and the Environment (NY: Vintage Books, 1998), 13. (To be cited as Steingraber #1)
[8] Colburn, 182.

Sidney Junior-Senior High School. Going from being the proverbial "big fish in a little pond" to a much larger "pond" did not seem to deter her. She continued to excel academically and socially. Soon, she became one of the leaders of her class, to be followed by recognition as one of the important student leaders of the entire school.

Becoming a cheerleader was one of Donna Jo's important goals – a goal she achieved with distinction. Looking prim and proper was another value. While it was permissible to launder the uniforms, Donna Jo insisted that hers be dry-cleaned. She did not know at the time that beginning the year before, another DDT-based chemical (perchlorethyline) had been authorized as a mothproofing agent in dry-cleaning.[9] However, if she had known in 1953 what became understood 46 years later, Donna Jo may very well have cared a great deal.

A 1999 Massachusetts Department of Public Health study found that 45% of those women in high breast cancer incidence areas of the city of Newton, used dry-cleaning services at least once per month, as compared to 32% for those in the less-affected sections of the city. Thus, the "miracle chemical" found one more pathway to the human body. Scientific ingenuity had ironically found a means, potentially, to cheerfully shorten a cheerleader's life.[10]

As if those exposures to DDT were not enough, there was more. Due to Mike and Donna Jo's residency in Washington, DC, often needing to return to Iowa to be with family; and due to Donna Jo's travels as a journalist, she would have been exposed numerous times to one other potentially lethal and foolhardy use of DDT. We do not know how often she may have been seated in the confines of a commercial airliner while a stewardess walked down the aisle spraying DDT to disinfect the craft, but it was a most common practice at the time.[11]

I am standing now at the memorial site Mike and his two sons erected for Donna Jo in the backyard. A large pink and white

---

[9] Steingraber #1, 7.

[10] www.usatoday.com/life/health/cancer/breast/hcbr041

[11] See "Photo Stories," July 12, 2002; www.beyondpesticides.org/photostories; see also https://www.dailytelegraph.com.au/news/nsw/landmark-legal-case-will-probe-the-link-between-parkinsons-disease-and-insecticide-sprays-used-on-longhaul-flights/news-story/8bed79471fc461cfaf1680ebc82265cf.

granite stone lies over the spot where her ashes are buried. A simple marker informs all who visit of the tragedy that has happened here. Ironically, Donna Jo's remains lie underneath the long-deceased grape arbor of her youth. Mike tells me that until her last breath, neither he, nor the boys were prepared for the shock of her departure.

Before leaving, I ask Mike if I can have one last look at the 1985 family portrait. Standing before that colorful portrayal of a very content and happy family, I am bewildered by the realization that it was only three years after the portrait was finished that it became known there was a significant statistical association between agricultural chemical use and cancer mortality.[12] Donna Jo died ten years later.

SANDRA (1955-2000)

March 2000: On my way to Sandra's home, I drive once again to Donna Jo's to see how Mike is doing now that considerable time has elapsed since her death. Since Sandra lives just over the hill from Mike, I have the greatest urge to ask if he knows anything about Sandra. However, that is something I cannot do. It would be a violation of patient confidentiality. After a short visit with Mike, I proceed on to Sandra's for one of my most challenging patient encounters.

Her smile lights up the room as if a floodlight came on. She has a way of making a stranger instantly feel welcome and at home in her presence. She is a large woman with a commanding presence. There is an engaging sparkle in her eyes, as if at any moment a burst of laughter might fill the room with merriment and joy. Today, however, there is little joy or merriment to be found. I am the hospice chaplain who has come to visit a 44-year-old woman who is dying of cancer – and that woman is Sandra.

While she knows she is dying, it is nearly impossible for her to admit that the end is within sight. Sandra speaks of wanting to be around for her three-year-old grandson, JD's, graduation from high school. She insists on doing one more cancer treatment, despite her physician's clear statement that her cancer is beyond cure. Death and

---

[12] A Study of 1497 US rural counties reported by: C.S. Stokes and K.D. Brace, "Agricultural Chemical Use and Cancer Mortality in Selected Rural Counties in the U.S.A," Journal of Rural Studies 4 (1988), 239-247.

preparing for death are beyond Sandra's ability to discuss just now. She lives somewhere between denial and avoidance.

Why talk about death when there is so much to live for? Why would she focus on planning a funeral when what she most desperately wants to do is get back to making lesson plans? Why talk about her future in the after-life when her greatest urge is to be back in the classroom with the children whom she loves?

Why talk about hope in the unseen when hope has already been shattered more than a few times? First, it was all the hopes and dreams she and Jim had for a long life together. But now a doctor has said "There is nothing more we can do."

Second, there were all the hopes and dreams she possessed about working with behaviorally disordered children—these dreams contained ways to break through the barriers and make a difference in those precious lives. But now she cannot get from bed to bathroom without help. There are moments when she admits to herself and others that the very idea of getting to her classroom wears her out, but the dream of being there energizes her.

Then, there are those twin questions again: "Why has this happened to me? What did I do wrong?" However, Sandra at first thought she knew why. It was after being hit by a book thrown by one of her students that the bruised breast, which never healed, was found to be cancerous.

She experiences a mixture of a fear of dying and a near-absolute refusal to let go. She is not sure there is a place to go after life on earth. Leaving a sure thing for the Great Unknown is not particularly appealing. However, the most compelling reasons to hang onto life are her lust for life and the whole disbelief that life can be so short.

On this unusually cold March day, Sandra's physician calls our office to say that he has about reached his limit with Sandra's repeated requests for more treatments and miracle cures. He wants hospice to talk to her and convince her that he is doing all he can do. It is my job now, along with Lisa, the RN, says our Executive Director, to convince Sandra that all anyone can do is to make her comfortable during her remaining days of life. This is not going to be an easy task, nor a pleasant one.

As a hospice chaplain, I try the usual approach of starting from where we know she is emotionally, acknowledging and affirming her well-known fears and wishes for a longer life. We allow Sandra all the time needed to cry and lament, vent and review all that has happened to her. The result? Well, Sandra asks her sister to get on the phone to make an appointment with her doctor and to "ask him to prescribe a new treatment for me."

When told that our presence at this very moment IS her doctor's prescription and that he has asked us to tell her he has done all he can do for her from a curative standpoint, Sandra becomes hysterical. "No, no, no! Don't tell me that! Don't tell me that! Dear God-in-Heaven, don't tell me that!!

We let her cry and cry she does. Great gushing sobs. Screams. Tears and groans. Finally, after what seemed at first to be an endless and relentless episode of profound fear, mixed with anger, Sandra takes possession of herself and says: "Thank you. I knew it all along. I just could not face it." The change in her demeanor and tone is sharp and sudden as switching off a hard rock CD in mid-track.

Two years after Sandra's death, I interviewed her two sisters. As we sat in her older sister's living room in the small town of Sidney, the County Seat of Fremont County, Sandra's story unfolded.

It was a stifling hot and humid hot day in 1955 when Sandra, the youngest of four children, joined the Johnson family on a Missouri River bottomland farm just over the bluff and west of Sidney. While she was 14 years younger than Donna Jo, and Donna Jo was out of high school before Sandra entered kindergarten, they had several things in common. They attended the same junior/senior high schools. They were both raised on a farm. Both were born prematurely; and while waging their final futile battles to stay alive, they were living less than one mile apart from each other.

However, these two girls had even more in common than all of that: Sandra, her siblings, and Donna Jo attended small rural schools where drinking water was supplied from adjacent wells. Both schools were surrounded by croplands. While Donna Jo's farm well was on higher ground than the Johnson well, both wells were in the direct downward flow from nearby higher croplands. It was the very summer of Sandra's birth that Donna Jo's mother closed-up the original well out of concern for its water quality and had another one dug further down the hill, but still in the cropland drainage basin.

In addition, the crop dusters swooping down over the fields fascinated Sandra, her siblings, and Donna Jo. It was mesmerizing to watch the chemicals fall from the planes and drift as if by their own will across the land. The roar of the planes spoke of power and control. The Johnson children and Donna Jo were also remotely united in their dislike for the taste that hung-on for hours, the lingering smell, and the burning sensation in their eyes afterward.

Cornfields sprayed with herbicides surrounded their homes and schools. When the fields were being sprayed from the air, "we were right in the middle of it," claims Sandra's younger sister who has withstood four cancer scares.

While Donna Jo could see as far as the end of the next section[13] to the north, and even as far as three sections to the west from her backyard, it was a limited view compared to Sandra's. The Johnson farm sat almost literally in the middle of the Missouri River bottomland. You can stand today in front of the abandoned foundation of the old homestead and, looking either to the west, the south, or the north, see the horizon stretch out almost endlessly. This land is as flat as flatland can ever become. To the east is another story, nearly the same, but different in that three sections away the flatness is abruptly interrupted by the Loess Hills bluffs that provide sanctuary for the village of Sidney.

I stand now beneath an old oak tree near where the family home once promised a bright future. All that is left are the vague outlines of the foundations for the house, one of the barns, and the well cover that is partially open and mostly worn away.
I imagine the Johnsons at work, at play, and a rest. The past is present:

Trees surround the house and outbuildings, providing shade and comfort from the sometimes-searing heat and stifling humidity on this Midwestern landscape. The well is a few feet from the house.

The well, however, is not well; in fact, this well is nearly terminal with its brackish color originating from the concentrated iron content of the soil through which the water travels. Thank God

---

[13] A section is one square mile.

for the Culligan Man! The family relies on the Culligan process for their cooking and drinking water. Yet, there are times when they have no choice but to use the well water for all purposes – at least for bathing, and least often for the family laundry. Washing clothes in this water is simply counter-productive.

Sandra and her sisters are about to enter the old chicken house that their father fixed up for the children as a playhouse. Sandra's older sister, Susan, is carrying the long-handled DDT spryer with the little glass jar containing the chemical at the end opposite the pump-handle. As she opens the door to the playhouse, she begins "fumigating the place" – an almost daily ritual in the summer to rid it of flies and crickets. As the spray settles, the children settle into their play-world.

Sandra's sister and brother, and Donna Jo had one other formative factor in common: they were all breast-fed by their mothers. Unfortunately, by 1950-51, three to four years prior to Sandra's birth and 12-years after Donna Jo's, significant concentrations of DDT had been discovered in human breast milk.[14]

If this had been acted upon in 1951 by a government concerned about the health of its people, rather than remaining confined to a publicly obscure scientific journal, could such regulatory action have made a difference? Would Sandra's sister have been spared the fear, four-times over, of an early death. Would the entire family have been spared the horror of watching Sandra die an early death?

Environmental factors were bad enough for Donna Jo, but they became much worse for Sandra. Five years before her birth, "Beech-Nut Packing Co., began allowing detectable levels of (pesticide) residue in baby food"[15]; the food of choice by Sandra's mother for her youngest. When Sandra was four-years-old in 1959, 80 million pounds of DDT were applied in the US alone, its peak usage.[16]

Sandra graduated from Sidney High School (as did Donna Jo), married, had two daughters, and became a very successful and well-liked teacher. In 1996 at the age of 41, Sandra was diagnosed with breast cancer. After enduring extremely painful and injurious

---

[14] Laug, et al., 245-46.
[15] Steingraber #1, 10.
[16] Regenstein, 338.

treatments for nearly three years, Sandra's cancer was believed to be in remission. Shortly after, the cancer was back with a vengeance and she died within three months – living at the time less than two miles from Donna Jo's farmstead.

We now know that Sandra experienced multiple exposures to DDT during her formative years. When she was 18-years-old, DDT was banned in the US (1973). We also know now, according to the 2010 President's Cancer Panel (PCP) Report, that:

Girls exposed to elevated levels of DDT before puberty (emphasis added), *when mammary cells are more susceptible to carcinogenic effects of chemicals, hormones, and radiation are five times more likely to develop breast cancer in middle age.*[17]

Sandra's mother, while providing much of the care during the last three months of Sandra's life, kept a well-guarded secret from her family. She, too, had been diagnosed with cancer. The fallout from Sandra's death and her mother's subsequent revelations was gravely devastating for the entire family. One year after Sandra's death, her mother attempted suicide.

JoAn (1958-2000)

September 2000: She is lying in her hospital bed, nearly blind from breast cancer gone rampant into her lungs and brain. She just celebrated her 42nd birthday and knows she will not celebrate another. Harley, her faithful black Rottweiller, lies at her bed side – until I step through the doorway. It is then that Harley rises and comes forward arching his body like a wall between this stranger and the object of his guardianship. JoAn speaks softly to Harley: "It's OK Harley." Harley resumes his reclining posture. "Since I have

---

[17] President's Cancer Panel, Environmental Cancer Risks: What We Can Do Now (2008-2009 Annual), US Department of Health and Human Services, National Institute of Health, National Cancer Institute, April 2010; citing B.A. Cohn, M.S. Wolff, P.M. Cirillo, and R.I. Sholtz, "DDT and breast cancer in young women: new data on the significance of age at exposure," Environmental Health Perspectives 2007; 115: 1406-14.

been pretty much confined to bed, this crazy dog rarely leaves this room. He takes good care of me," JoAn says, choking back the tears.

The tumors in and around the lungs are choking off life-giving oxygen. Tumors in the brain have already destroyed much of her sight. Now those tumors are eroding her ability to speak.

She is exhausted. When she tries to speak, words fail to form. Thoughts are left dangling, both in the air and in her mind. There is little more communication to be had between us. She is beyond a readiness to die. JoAn simply wants to be done with it.

Suddenly, Harley stands up and comes forward, pressing against me. It is amazing! This dog is telling me my time is up. However, JoAn says, haltingly, "Would you pray with me?" As I begin with the prayer, Harley returns to his reclining position. At the "Amen", he rises again and pushes me toward the door.

Then, just as I am about to honor Harley's invitation to leave, I hear the so very common and heart-ripping double-barreled inquiry once again: "Why has this happened to me? What did I do wrong."

While walking out onto JoAn's front porch, I hesitate for a moment as I realize her home is but blocks away from Sandra's family home after they moved off the farm. Furthermore, if it were not for the trees, I could see Donna Jo's farm home from this spot.

Sometime after JoAn's death, I was granted the opportunity to interview her husband Jim and his mother. Their understanding of JoAn's history is most enlightening:

∎∎∎

It was a bitterly cold and blustery day in January 1958 when JoAn was born into a farm family trying to make ends meet on bottomland property. Like Sandra and Donna Jo, JoAn was breast fed as an infant, raised on well-water both at home and at school, and joyously romped in the sprays of the crop duster bi-planes flying over the fields.

JoAn, like Sandra, was also raised on Beech Nut Packing Company's baby food with the distinctive small squat bottles and a happy contented smiling baby peering from the label. Donna Jo, being older, missed the Beech Nut nutritional program; perhaps it was just as well.

Within a decade of DDT's introduction into American life, its deadly presence expanded from the air one breathes, to drinking water, to the food supply, to mothers' milk, to the "sanitized" food for "Healthy, Happy Babies." And Paul Muller won the Nobel Prize for its development.[18]

Before JoAn dies, she witnesses two sisters, two aunts and an uncle die from cancer – all of whom were born and raised in the same location as JoAn. All would have been exposed to the same environmental factors, not least of which were the facts that by 1959:

- *Geigy Chemical Company's sale of the new pesticides atrazine and simazine begins to rise from 15,890 pounds in '59 to 64 million pounds in '69 with a $90 million profit.[19]*
- *Crops treated with pesticides in the US begin to increase from 20% of the total in '59 to 96% in '88.[20]*
- A year later, herbicide use commences its own dramatic increase by 800% into the 1980's.[21]

In 1962, when one out of fourteen American women were at risk of having breast cancer, Rachel Carson published her controversial book, Silent Spring,[22] warning of the effects of DDT and other chemicals on the environment, plant, animal, fish, bird and human life. By then Donna Jo was 22 years old, Sandra 7, JoAn 4, and Susan (whom we shall soon meet) was a rambunctious 3-year-old.

JoAn married, had a family, divorced, and remarried. In hindsight, according to Jim, the signs of cancer were evident as early a 1992 when she began experiencing un-accounted-for pain. She was 34-years-old. It was nearly 8 years later when JoAn was diagnosed with lung and breast cancer metastasizing to the brain.

---

[18] Colburn, 69.

[19] Dan Fagan, Marianne Lavalle, and the Center for Public Integrity, Toxic DeceptionL How the Chemical Industry Manipulates Science, Bends the Law, and Endangers Your Health, (Secaucus, NJ: Carol Publishing Group, 1996), 18.

[20] Lo.cit.

[21] William A. Battaglin, Earl M. Thurman, Stephen J. Kalkhoff, and Steven D. Porter," Herbicides and Transformation Products in Surface Waters of the Midwestern United States, Journal of the American Water Resources Association, August 2003, 743.

[22] Rachel Carson, Silent Spring, (Boston: Houghton Mifflin, 1962).

The family was gathered in the living room one day in September 2000, when they noticed Harley leaving JoAn's bedroom with head drooping. It was then that they knew JoAn had died.

Harley, previously, a perfectly healthy dog, died 3 months later from an apparent broken heart.

SUSAN (1959-2000)

October 2000: She is just getting home as I arrive at her rented farmhouse. While she had not been feeling well for some time, she had been informed only 48 hours earlier that she has inoperable and untreatable cancer throughout her body. Every nodal system is infected with the dreaded disease. Jacob, her 12-year-old son is helping his mother make the slow journey from car to house. Her sister, the driver remains in the car, weeping. The look on Jacob's face is that of an old man who has decided the dreams of youth are utter folly.

Susan is angry at the disease. She is angry at the unknown cause, and she too asks, as so many do, "Why has this happened to me? What did I do wrong? She is angry with the doctors who say, "There is nothing more we can do." From her perspective, the doctors **NEVER** did anything, except abandon her. Finally, she is angry at the prospect of not being around to see Jacob grow to maturity. She wants so much to see him become proficient on that trombone—the instrument she always dreamed of playing, but had to give up, due to family financial circumstances when she was his age.

The problem of family financial insecurity is one that has haunted Susan all her life and is one that is about to raise its ugly head once again in a devastating manner. Within three days after her admission to hospice care, Susan and her husband are informed of their eviction. They have 10 days to move out. Given the need to find another home, pack up and move out of one place into another, transferring Susan to the local nursing home is the only solution to the all-important issue of providing adequate and consistent care.

Lola, Susan's mother, claims that it was the day when our hospice staff assisted in Susan's transfer to the nursing home that she experienced the saddest and most heartbreaking day of her life. As parents, we do not anticipate living to see our child admitted to a nursing home, to say nothing of that child dying before us. But, that was Lola's lot in life. Susan died three weeks later.

A while after Susan's death, her mother granted me a lengthy interview filling me in on many of the details of Susan's life:

****

On April 13, 1972, Susan's 13th birthday, she and her parents moved to a farm one-mile from the small Iowa town of Farragut. While most of the buildings are gone today, it is a beautiful spot with huge oak trees surrounding what once were the farmhouse, barn and other outbuildings. All that remain today are a shed and the water pump above the well.

"When it rained," according to Lola, "the water would stream off the fields and head right for that well." She recalls workers spreading fertilizer and spraying pesticides, then coming to the house for lunch and stopping at the well to wash up—rinsing directly into the open well. "The chemicals," Lola claims, are responsible for her daughter's premature death, as well as the death of many others in this valley. "Everyone knows it," she adds. And the words of the Leonard Cohen song, *Everybody Knows* come to mind.

Soon after Susan's 13th birthday in 1972, DDT is officially banned from use in the US. But the rise in incidence of cancer in Iowa increases by 26% for males and 37% for females between 1973 and 1998,[23] while breast cancer incidence increases nationally by 40% during the same period of time.[24] The lower Nishnabotna Valley would suffer a 41% increase in cancer-related deaths over roughly the same space of time, while the State of Iowa experiences a 20% average increase.[25] Simply having been born in this area of Iowa brings with it a doubling of the likelihood of contracting and dying of cancer. In addition, we would learn later that between 1970 and 1994 brain cancer, leukemia, Hodgkin's & Non-Hodgkin's deaths would rank higher in the Midwest than in any other areas in the US.[26]

---

[23] Cancer Registry of Iowa – 2001 Cancer Report (University of Iowa), 6.

[24] American Cancer Society, "Annual Report Shows Overall Decline in US Cancer Incidence and Death Rates," June 5, 2001 (Atlanta, GA) www.cancer.org/docroot/MED/content/MED21xAnnualReportShowsOverall.

[25] Willis Goudy, Sandra Chawat Burke, and Margaret Hansen, Iowa's Counties: Selected Population Trends, Vital Statistics and Socioeconomic Data (Census Service, Department of Sociology, Iowa State University, October 2000), 122-125.

[26] Lynn R. Goldman, Geographic Analysis: Cancer Mortality Maps, US, 1970-1994, 5-8.

It is into these times and these circumstances that all four of these women were born and raised. These were their formative years. It is here in Fremont County that their hopes and dreams were nourished. Visions of love, marriage, family, and careers sprouted and were cultivated from this geography of the soul.

It would take another decade before federal and state governments would initiate databases known as Cancer Registries. In the meantime, between 1965 and 1970 the average human intake of DDT is estimated to have been 23 times higher than in 1982.[27]

Suppose for a moment: If Hueper & Conway's 1964 warning of "a cancer...epidemic...(fueled by) chemical and physical carcinogens"[28] had been acted upon in 1964 rather in 1972, would it have made a difference in five-year-old Susan's life? Or, in 24-year-old Donna Jo's life?

Instead of any preventative or precautionary measures being taken, Monsanto Corporation in 1969 introduced alachlor, which becomes the "key ingredient for Lasso, Bronco, Bullet, CANNON, Freedom and Lariat."[29] All are destined to become products of choice throughout the country for eradicating weeds from croplands.

In 1971, a "War on Cancer" is declared by President Richard M. Nixon, ultimately leading to the enactment of the 1974 Federal Safe Drinking Water Act, enabling the creation of rural water treatment facilities. Five years later, in 1979, rural water treatment facilities come to the Midwest. However, by now Donna Jo is 39 years, Sandra is 24, JoAn is 21, and Susan is 20. The damage is already done and, according to Lola, "Everybody knows!"

In 1974, the very same year Congress promulgated the Safe Drinking Water Act, scientists were discovering chlorination byproducts (CBPs) in public waters.[30] According to Edstrom Industries, an agricultural research and development firm, CBPs such as chloroform, bromodichloromethane, chlorodibromomethane, dichloroacetic acid, and trichloroacetic acid cause liver and kidney

---

[27] Steingraber #1, 169.

[28] CF 6.

[29] Fagan, 22.

[30] Consider the Source: Farm Runoff, Chlorination By-Products, and Human Health (Environmental Working Group [U.S. PIRG], 202), 21.

tumors in rats and mice.[31] The Human Health and Great Lakes Division of the Great Lakes Commission, an interstate compact[32], reports "(e)vidence from toxicologic and epidemiologic studies suggest a link between by-products of the chlorination process and increased risk of some cancers (e.g., bladder and colon) and adverse pregnancy outcomes (e.g., miscarriage, birth defects and low birth weight)."[33]

Congress, however, from 1979 to 2002 exempted small water suppliers (serving <10,000 people) from testing for CBPs.[34] In 1984, five years after federally-funded rural water treatment facilities came to the Midwest, most of the towns in Fremont County, indeed throughout most of the corn belt, remained exempt from testing for CBPs. Yet, research reported from Italy that year had established links between farm-women's exposure to herbicides such as atrazine and subsequent diagnoses of ovarian cancer.[35]

Four years after the Italian report, the American study by Stokes and Brace indicated a strong relationship between chemical use and cancer mortality.[36] In 1989, a year after the Stokes & Brace findings were reported, other startling findings were reported: Atrazine was found to exist in 93% of Iowa water samples,[37] and 98% of Midwest watershed streams and rivers had "detectable levels of…atrazine, metolachlor, and alachlor after spring and summer rain storms."[38]

---

[31] www.edstrom.com/resources.

[32] The Great Lakes Commission des Grans Lacs is composed of the eight Great Lakes US States (NY, PA, OH, IL, IN, WS, MI, & MN) as well as the Canadian Provinces of Ontario and Quebec who are associate members. The GLC "promotes the orderly, integrated and comprehensive development, use and conservation of water and related resources of the Great Lakes Basin and St. Lawrence River." See: www.glc.org/about.

[33] www.great-lakes.net/humanhealth/other/chlorine.

[34] Loc. Cit.

[35] A. Donna, et al., "Ovarian Mesothlial Tumors and Herbicides: A Case-Control Study," Carcinogenesis 5 (1984): 941-942.

[36] CF# 10.

[37] John Wargo, Our Children's Toxic Legacy: How Science & Law Fail to Protect Us from Pesticides (Yale University Press, 1996), 12.

[38] Iowa Association of Naturalists, "Iowa Agricultural Practices & the Environment," Iowa Environmental Issues Series (Sept 19980, 8.

Unfortunately, 20 years later (2009) a NY Times article announced that "Millions in U.S. Drink Dirty Water."[39] If only the water was simply "dirty". The facts, as reported, were that "over three million Americans have been exposed since 2005 to drinking water with illegal concentrations" of chemicals. To Donna Jo, Sandra, JoAn, and Susan, their families and friends, all these studies did not matter. It was simply too late.

A few weeks before her death, I was privileged to be with Susan and her family. I invited them all, her husband, son, mother and a friend, to join in prayer around Susan and to say what they needed to say to her and about her.

After the session ended, I walked out onto the front porch. As I looked across the valley with its prosperous croplands and undulating hills, I was struck by a profound and numbing realization that I could see from there Donna Jo's farm, Sandra's home, as well as JoAn's. And I wondered aloud to myself, "What is going on here?" Well, I knew what was going on. Young women were dying. The real question was WHY?

Already in 2000, I knew some of the reasons for those young women's deaths. For example, I had learned that twenty years before then in 1980, Dr. Melvin Reuber was fired from his job as Director of Experimental Pathology Laboratory at the Frederick (Maryland) Cancer Research Center for questioning the findings and procedures of pesticide studies funded by chemical companies. In addition, the very same year that Susan, JoAn and Sandra died (2000), I had seen a news report concerning the firing of Dr. Omar Shafey. He lost his job with the Florida Department of Health, apparently for refusing to soften his research conclusions that pesticide spraying is harmful to public health (see Chapter Seven: "Cooptation: Expertise vs. Collusion.").

The system had conspired against these women and countless others, as well as against those like Reuber, Shafey and others like them who were simply trying to tell the truth.

---

[39] Charles Duhigg, "Millions in U.S. Drink Dirty Water, Records Show," NY Times (December 8, 2009).

Chapter Two

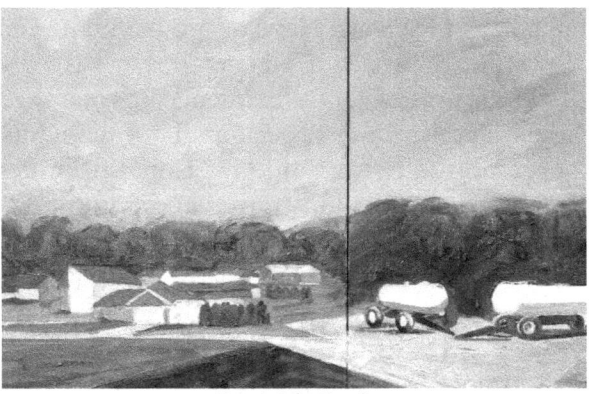

Pesticide Tanks

Chemical Warfare and Pacification:
The Parallels in American Agricultural and Military Policies

Body Counts

At first, it seemed we, as a hospice, were dealing with a cancer cluster in southwest Iowa. Research, however, took a somewhat surprising turn. The problem is not isolated to the Nishna Valley. It also lies with the Des Moines River Valley and the Big Spring Basin in Iowa. It extends from Iowa to the Platte, Elkhorn & Niobrara River Valleys in Nebraska. It lurks in every Corn Belt state. Nor is it unique to young women. We observe it in the cancer-related deaths record for older women, men and children. It haunts the cranberry bogs of Cape cod, Massachusetts, and lies along the Hudson River Valley, the San Luis Valley of South-Central Colorado, the Rio Grande Valley of New Mexico. In fact, the problem of chemically induced cancer exists everywhere and anywhere pesticides are used whether it is in Canada, Colombia, India, Malaysia, France, or Germany, to name but a few.

September 11, 2001 has become a new "Day of Infamy." With the death toll at nearly 3000 civilians, the "Attack on America" surpasses Pearl Harbor on December 7, 1941, in its horror, treachery, and devastation to property and human lives. As horrifying as Pearl Harbor and the entire war were, the ending of World War II only seems to have ushered-in a period of even greater destruction of human lives.

With the end of the war came the need to find peacetime uses for the chemicals and technologies devised to wage war. With the end of the war against Fascism, Nazism and Totalitarianism, there emerged a new kind of war – a war against a sustainable society. Growth, production, profits, and abundance (as well as consequent scarcity[40] where bigger is better), became the trademarks of success; indeed, they became the bottom line measures of American policy whether foreign or domestic, industrial or agricultural.

As World War II ended with the dropping of "Little Boy" by the Enola Gay on Hiroshima on August 6, 1945, and "Fat Man" on Nagasaki three days later, it was as if the radioactive mushroom clouds over those faraway cities drifted invisibly and noiselessly across the ocean and back to the "Heartland of America" where the Enola Gay had, so to speak, been born. The Enola Gay originated from Bellevue, Nebraska, no more than 30 miles, as the crow flies, from Sidney, Iowa.

The Donna Jos of Heartland America were at ground zero and, in a figurative sense, should have seen it coming; but then, so too, should the Marias and Estellas who lived in the Rio Grande Valley of New Mexico near Los Alamos, the very birthplace of the Atomic bomb -- not to mention Almagordo's White Sands Atomic Testing Grounds.

Perhaps it is safe to say that humankind's participation in WWII, the development of atomic and chemical war technology, the harnessing of that same know-how to the land in so-called peacetime with consequent effects upon human health, all provide proof of author and retired Presbyterian pastor Marv Hiles' theory of the futility of war:

War may be executed with brilliant plans, but at some point, physically, it goes awry. There is a beast in us that roams this way and that, driven not by plans but by base instincts.[41]

One might say the "chickens have come home to roost." The atomic bomb unleashed a chemical war on a way of life and a quality

---

[40] "Human Development: Abundance and Scarcity – A Pastoral Letter on the Economy of Northeast Nebraska," by Archbishop Daniel Sheehan, Archdiocese of Omaha, January 11, 1991

[41] Marv Hiles, The Way Through: Contemplative Companion (#14) Late Autumn, 2003.

of life in rural America. The Donna Jo's in this world are living with it, suffering and dying from it.

The American Cancer Society estimates 547,000 Americans died from cancer in 1995.[42] In Iowa , the cancer body count from 1974 to 1998 came to 59,000 people[43] -- a loss of life greater than the 58,169 American deaths sustained in the Vietnam War.[44] In 1995 1.2 million people in the U.S. were told they had cancer – that is 3,400 people per day (142 per hour, and over 2 per minute) being faced with a life threatening attack.[45] All of this is background to the environment in which Donna Jo, Sandra, JoAn and Susan lived and died.

While the breast cancer death rate has been declining by an estimated two percent yearly since 1990, by 2004 approximately 2.4 million women living in the US had a history of breast cancer.[46] In addition, Science Daily reported in 2009 that "cancer incidence rates continue to grow,"[47] an observation supported by the President's Cancer Panel in 2010:

In 2009 alone, approximately 1.5 million men, women, and children were diagnosed with cancer, and 562,000 died from the disease.[48]

Donna Jo, Sandra, JoAn, and Susan are members of what Sandra Steingraber, Ph.D., an ecologist and cancer survivor, believes to be "the most poisoned generation to come of adult age."[49] The simple fact is as a society we did not, at the time, know what is known now. But we had been warned.

---

[42] The Universal Almanac 1996.

[43] Goudy, 121.

[44] www.militaryfactory.com/American_War_deaths.asp.

[45] Steingraber #1, 32.

[46] American Cancer Society, "American Cancer Society Report Finds breast Cancer Death Rate Continues to Drop," (September 25, 2007) www.cancer.org/docroot/MED.

[47] Van Andel Research Institute (2009, August 14). "Cancer Mortality Rates Experience Steady Decline: conventional Method May Underreport Declining Death Rate for All Age Groups." Science Daily Retrieved February 13, 2010 http://www.sciencedaily.com/releases/2009/08/090813142359.htm.

[48] PCP 2010, Cover Letter to President Barak Obama, signed by LaSalle D. Leffall, Jr., MD, Chair, and Margaret L. Kripke, Ph.D.

[49] Steingraber #1, 115.

When Donna Jo was four years-old (1945), 10 years before Sandra was born, and 13 years before JoAn entered this world, the Fish and Wildlife Service (FWS) issued a DDT alarm. In a press release issued on August 22, 1945, the FWS described the results of DDT tests "warning that the pesticide should be used with extreme caution," and anyone observing 'unusual reactions' in wildlife following an exposure to DDT…" should "report it at once."[50]

This warning was preceded by an even more chilling alarm on August 10, 1945 by a young FWS employee by the name of Rachel Carson. In her memo to fish processing plant operators, Carson warned of the "potential hazards of using DDT in their facilities (and) preliminary experiments indicated that DDT was toxic to animals and humans when ingested…."[51]

Despite these early warnings, it seemed too preposterous to think that these chemicals would even be allowed on the market, if they were harmful to human health. But, it was clear from the labels and slick advertisements that, while one needed to be careful in their use, the products were safe, helpful, effective—and "productive." What more did we need?

American Agricultural Policy

This was the beginning of our modern era of American agriculture with its emphasis on production and expansion where bigger is considered better and using food as a foreign policy weapon. These policies encouraged a movement to larger-and-larger farm holdings with ready availability of bank loans to buy land, equipment, seeds, fertilizer, and pesticides. None of the families represented here survived as farm families. Donna Jo's husband continued, after her death, living on the property without actually farming. All four families, in a real sense, have been effectively displaced – victims of the "commercial conquest"[52] of family farming.

---

[50] William Souder, On a Further Shore: The Life and Legacy of Rachel Carson (NY: Crown Publishers, 2012), 8; citing U.S. Fish and wildlife Service Press Release, Aug 22, 1945, NCTC, National Conservation Training Center Museum and Archives, Shepherdstown, WV.
[51] Souder, 113.
[52] Wendell Berry, The Unsettling of America Culture & Agriculture (NY: Avon, 1978, 6.

Fremont County, Iowa, mirrors the familiar image of family farming across the US since the early 1980's. The total number of farms decreased from 771 in 1982 to 568 in 1997; yet:

- The total acreage being farmed increased by nearly 12,000, the equivalent of 20 square miles.
- The average farm acreage increased from 398 to 560.
- The number of 1,000+ acre farms increased from 51 to 102.
- The number of farms with fewer than 50 acres dropped from 213 to 62; and finally:
- The total number of farms producing a value of sales less than $10,000/year decreased by 60% (from 90 to 54).
- Those bringing in less than $50,000/year decreased by 44% (from 280 to 123), and the number of farms producing sales of $100,000 or more increased by 35% (from 178 to 240).[53]

Caveat # 3: Having said all this, let us be mindful that world-wide we have a picture that is at once similar and different. The Food and Agriculture Organization (FAO) reports that "About 70 percent of the food we consume globally comes from smallholder farmers."[54] Yet, the FAO notes that "small farms occupy less than a quarter of agricultural land, and the holdings are getting smaller."[55]

Small-scale farmers, particularly women, are the backbone of agricultural production worldwide. They produce 70 percent of the food consumed in Africa on less than 15 percent of available

---

[53] Department of Economics, Iowa State University, "Census of Agriculture-Fremont County," *Iowa Profiles: Public Resources Online*(Ames: ISU, September 1998) www.profiles.iastate.edu/data/census/county/agcensus.asp?sCounty=19071.

[54] Meriel Watts and Stephanie Williamson, "Executive Summary: Replacing Chemicals with Biology: Phasing out Highly Hazardous Pesticides with Agroecology(Pesticide Action Network International, Penang, Malaysia, 2015), 10. www.panap.net/sites/default/files/Phasing-Out-HHPs-with-Agroecology.pdf.

[55] Ibid, 10, citing GRAIN, 2014. "Hungry for Land: Small farmers feed the world with less than a quarter of all farmland," http://www.grain.

agricultural land; in sub-Saharan Africa and in Asia that figure rises to 80 percent.[56]

Emphasis then shifted to higher yields for export to the international market, and financial incentives changed as well. The "smart money" now was in having the land, tools, and resources to produce, produce, and produce. The only way to survive was to borrow from the banks, expand farm operations, and exploit the land by using every square foot of the soil, and eradicate everything that could possibly stand in the way of the god of production.

As early as 1978 Wendell Berry warned that "exclusive emphasis on production will accelerate the mechanization and chemicalization of farming, increase the price of land, increase overhead and operating costs, and thereby diminish the farm population…."[57] Or, as Pope Francis states in his 2015 encyclical on the environment, in addressing many of the pollutants in the environment:

Substances which contribute to the acidification of soil and water, (are) fertilizers, insecticides, fungicides, herbicides and agrotoxins in general. Technology, which linked to business interests, is presented as the only way of solving these problems, in fact proves incapable of seeing the mysterious network of relations between things and so sometimes solves one problem only to create others.[58]

American Military & Agricultural Policy:
The Parallels & The Quest for Control

During the middle 1960's and 1970's American military policy in Vietnam used napalm and Agent Orange to defoliate forests and crops depriving the targeted enemy of food and cover. Little apparent regard was given for the effect upon our own military personnel, to say nothing of the long-term effects on the land and people of Vietnam.

---

[56] Ibid, 184.

[57] Wendell Berry, 10.

[58] Pope Francis, Laudato Si: On Care for Our Common Home (Vatican Press, May 24, 2015), 20.

At roughly the same time, American domestic agricultural policy encouraged widespread use of chemicals to increase crop production. Little apparent regard was given, however, for the impact of those chemicals upon the land or those sentient beings who inhabit it. Marty Strange, the founder of a rural advocacy organization, The Center for Rural Affairs based in Nebraska, observed in 1988:

> *The powerful, mysterious technology that fosters industrial agribusiness is directed at immediate materialistic objectives – more food and more profit – with little concern for long-run sustainability. If a technique can make twice the corn for one farm or farmer, it must be used, even if it eventually ruins both the farmer and the farm.*[59]

Also, during the 1960's – 1970's, US military strategy attempted to "pacify" entire villages in Vietnam, seeking to isolate the Vietcong. Whole populations were uprooted in a failed attempt to concentrate American control through relocation while reducing the Vietcong's control. Meanwhile, at home, American agricultural policy was heedlessly already responsible for uprooting thousands of families from their ancestral lands – a program that would lead to the concentration of farmland into the hands of the few.[60]

An extrapolation of the data noted earlier suggests that 203 Iowa families were displaced from their land between 1982 and 1997.[61] Put another way, that means it was 13 families/year leaving their farms and, in many cases, leaving their ancestral heritages behind.

As a society, the American people are, in a sense, victims of pacification. We have accepted the Madison Avenue sales pitch of a better life through the use and consumption of chemicals. As Wendel Berry has claimed:

> *If there is any law that has been consistently operative in American history, it is that the members of any established people or*

---

[59] Marty Strange, Family Farming: A New Economic Vision (Lincoln: University of Nebraska Press, 1988), 209.
[60] Wendell Berry, 10.
[61] See CF 53.

group or community, sooner or later become "redskins" – that is, they become the designated victims of an utterly ruthless, officially sanctioned and subsidized exploitation.[62]

Furthermore, in the last 30 years since 1988, the unfolding of unmitigated power and control over US (and international) agriculture and agricultural production by corporate farms, corporate chemical companies, and corporate seed companies has become a political, social, economic and medical plague.

Yes, a "War on Cancer" was declared in 1972, but the "battlefield conditions" are complicated due to multiple factors, namely (but not limited to) the following:

- Relentlessness of the Causes and of time itself
- Multiplicity of causes
- Ambiguities in environmental monitoring
- Individual, community, political and medical denial
- Collusion and complicity
- Readiness of victims to accept blame, and
- Preoccupation with downstream symptoms vs, upstream precipitators.

Each of these factors, and the element of denial inherent in each, will be examined here as we go forward. However, before doing so, another caveat of sorts, would be warranted:

The title of this chapter uses the phrase, *Chemical Warfare.* As we proceed through this book, it is hoped that the purpose in employing the concept of "war" is clear. However, we must be mindful of the caution brought forth by Albuquerque, New Mexico, journalist Winthrop Quigley:

"War" might be the most overused and most sloppily used word in American public life, and because it is we end up with sloppy thinking and poor public policies. Politicians have declared war on drugs, war on poverty, war on cancer.... As a rhetorical device, the

---

[62] Wendell Berry, 4 (emphasis in original). See also, Jacob Hacker & Paul Pierson, <u>Winner-Take-All Politics: How Washington Made the Rich Richer-And Turned Its Back on the Middle Class</u> (NY: Simon & Schuster, 2010.)

word "War" has its uses. It emphasizes the importance of the cause. It carries with it a sense of urgency, even crisis....[63]

The intent in using the notion of "Chemical warfare on our own people" is to not use it sloppily, but to employ the term with the best of intentions, emphasizing the urgency in stopping what constitutes avoidable death and human suffering.

---

[63] Winthrop Quigley, "The Word 'War' is a rhetorical minefield," Albuquerque Journal, December 10, 2015, 1 & 3.

Chapter Three

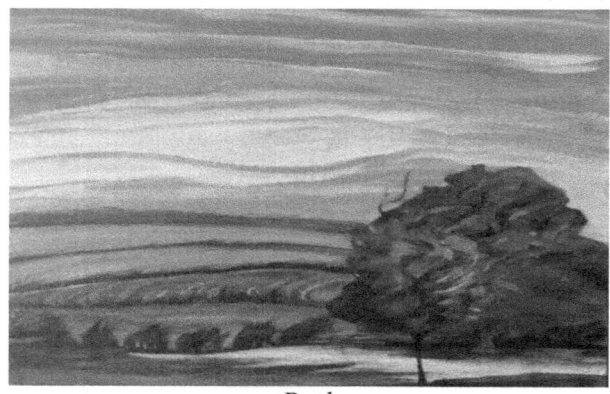

Dusk

Relentlessness of Causes and of Time:
Source-Points for Sickness & Pesticide Perdurability

Poisoning from exposure to pesticides is a problem the world over, but most especially in developing countries and most especially for women. Acute poisoning kills, maims or debilitates many millions of women every year.[64]
(Meriel Watts, Ph.D., New Zealand)

Assuming the exposure to DDT ingested from their mothers' milk, pesticides sprayed by planes, or chemicals running off from cropland into water wells at homes and schools, the "Donna Jos" were living with a life-threatening cancer clock that unrelentingly continued to tick. They were doomed eventually to early deaths by a preventable disease. Or, as the President's Cancer Panel reported to President Obama:

With the growing body of evidence linking environmental exposures to cancer, the public is becoming increasingly aware of the unacceptable burden of cancer resulting from environmental and

---

[64] Meriel Watts, Ph.D., <u>Pesticides & Breast Cancer: A Wake Up Call</u> (Penang, Malaysia: Pesticide Action Network [PAN Asia & the Pacific], 2007), 9.

occupational exposures that could have been prevented through appropriate national action.[65]

Signs of the Times: Source Points for Sickness

Ten to twenty years (1989-1999) years after federally-funded rural water treatment plants became fixtures of American life (1979), repeated studies by multiple agencies were reporting the magnitude of the consequences of the use of chemicals in the corporate drive to industrialize agriculture:

- The US Geological Survey found in a study conducted between 1989-1994 that atrazine was detected "in 990 of the 1604 water treatment samples drawn from Midwestern streams, rivers, reservoirs, and aquifers…" and in Iowa even rain drops were found to have excessive concentrations of the same pesticide.[66]
- An analysis of data obtained from the National Pesticide Use Database housed at the National Center for Food and Agricultural Policy (NCFAP) reveals the following truths:
  1. From 1992-1997 the average pounds per acre applied of the following chemicals:
     a. 2-4D
     b. Alachlor
     c. Atrazine, and
     d. Metolochlor
  2. Increased in Iowa, Nebraska, and Colorado
  3. While decreasing over-all only in New Mexico; yet,
  4. New Mexico's use of alachlor and metolochlor increased along with the other states.[67]
- A 1992 U.S. General Accounting Office report estimated that "as many as 300,000 farmworkers are poisoned by pesticides each year."[68]

---

[65] PCP 2010, Cover Letter.
[66] Steingraber #1, 20.
[67] www.cipm.ncsu.edu/croplife/getOutput.cfm.
[68] *The Use of Pesticides in New Mexico* www.farmworkers.org/pestieng

- In a 1992-1995 USGS study of the converging Platte and Elkhorn Valleys in Nebraska, it was disclosed that "herbicide loads increase with distance downstream."[69] Imagine what happens with the herbicide loads as all the Mississippi and Missouri rivers converge into the Gulf of Mexico.

- The herbicide and nitrate load accumulates as the ditches flow into the streams and creeks, and as the creeks flow into the rivers. As the rivers flow into the Gulf they produce a "hypoxic zone" *–the Dead Zone.*

- The Dead Zone occurs as the nutrients pouring into the Gulf spur the growth of "enormous algae blooms at the surface. The algae die, then settle to the bottom and decompose. This process uses up the dissolved oxygen in the lower depths and leaves too little oxygen for most aquatic species to survive."[70]

Time Marches On: Pesticide Perdurability

The process of degrading both the environment and human health appear to have no end in sight. Even more disturbing is the fact that it seems to take 10-20 years of research before we learn the environmental, toxicological and epidemiological consequences of our actions; and another 10-20 years before we do anything about it!

There simply is no magical solution to pollution. Even the enactment, for example, by the Nebraska State Unicameral Legislature in 1969 authorizing the creation of Natural Resource Districts (NRDs), designed to protect the integrity of water and land resources,[71] did not provide an immediate cure for the disease of the land and its water. It was not until 1986 for regulating agencies with special legal powers (Special Natural Resource Districts, SNRDs), monitoring areas of high nitrate/pesticide impact, to be authorized. It

---

[69] USGS, Water Quality in the Central Nebraska Basins, Nebraska, 1992-1995 www.water.usgs.gov/pub/circ1163, (updated September 14, 1998, 2) {to be cited here after as *Water Quality in Central Nebraska Basins.*

[70] *Earth & Sky*, November 27, 2001, (authored by Eleanor Imster & narrated by Joel Bloch and Debra Bird). www.earthsky,com/Shows.

[71] *The Upper Elkhorn Natural Resources District,* www.uenrd.org.

took four more years (1990) before the first Special Protection Area (SPA) was established in Nebraska.[72]

Assuming each step as required by law takes the maximum time allowed to come to completion, it may take as long as 591 days before regulations are in place ready to be enforced. That is one year and 7.5 months.[73] And time marches on. With it comes on-going human exposure. Even with the establishment of NRDs and with the strictest enforcement of Best Management Practices (BMPs), as well as maximum cooperation of all farmers and pesticide/nitrate applicators, no one knows how long it will take to detoxify the land and ground water.

According to the Colorado Department of Health and Environment's Water Quality Control Division, the San Luis Valley (SLV) of south-central Colorado is not immune to this problem. Since the "mainstream of the Rio Grande, as well as ground water within the San Luis Valley are used heavily for agriculture … nutrients such as ammonia and nitrates increase in concentration in this area."[74] Time, indeed, marches on, chemicals accumulate, cancers grow, people die, and families grieve. The sacrifice of human lives is laid upon the altar in worship to the Great God of Production; and "Everybody Knows."

****

JoAn: Surrounded by the Enemy and Running Out of Time

1992:
JoAn's cancer did not wait for a local NRD to begin regulating pesticide use, or for all farmers in the area to follow the very Best Management Practices. JoAn's cancer did not wait for that unknown, perhaps impossible, time when all the contaminants in the ground would disappear. JoAn's cancer did not retreat on her 14th birthday

---

[72] See Montgomery County, Maryland, *Special Protection Areas, www.montgomerycountymd.gov/deptmpl*, and North Carolina Cooperative Extension Service, *NWQEP Notes: The NCSU (North Carolina State University) Water Quality Group Newsletter,* July 1993, #60," www.bae.ncsu.edu/programs/extension/wqg/issuees/60.

[73] J. David Aiken, Special Ground Water Quality Protection Areas (Lincoln: University of Nebraska, January 1992).

[74] Water Quality in Colorado, 2000 (Water Quality Control Division, Colorado Department of Health and Environment).

when DDT was banned by the US Government, nor did her cancer panic and run for cover when the EPA ruled that pesticide applicators were required to be trained, certified, and licensed.[75] Rather there is every reason to believe her cancer matured as she did.

There is every reason, as well, to believe the very milk from her mother's breasts, the water she drank frim the farmstead's well and later at school, the food she ate from the garden, the air she breathed, and perhaps the clothes she wore, all contributed to the formation of the enemy within her body. And so it was, that one day in 1992, at the young age of 34, we can imagine a stabbing pain suddenly striking JoAn in her chest as she is assisting in the transfer of a nursing home resident from his wheel chair to the bed. At first she thinks she has strained a muscle.

Mary, the other nursing assistant, hears JoA's groan and asks, "What's going on JoAn?"

"Oh, nothing. Just twisted something. I'll be OK."

"Yeah, well, you sure don't look OK."

With that, JoAn suddenly feels nauseous and runs to the bathroom. It is a "false alarm" and soon she is feeling better.

But JoAn never gets better. However, it takes six years before she will be diagnosed with cancer. Six years of episodes similar to the one at the nursing home that day; six years of sometimes utterly immobilizing pain; six years of absolutely draining bouts of nausea; six years of trips to the ER; six years of x-rays, CT-scans, MRIs; six years of being told there is "nothing wrong"; six years of occasionally thinking she is "going crazy." How else could one explain her experiences?

"All of these doctors and all of the tests can't be wrong, for God's sake!" she rants one evening slamming her fist on the table. This outburst catches her husband, Jim, by surprise. He thought they were talking about their day – hers at the nursing home, his at the office.

While Jim understands what she is saying, and while he certainly knows the subject well, he is aghast at the sudden blast of anger. JoAn has always taken things in stride. Nothing has ever seemed to rile her. Jim does not recognize this woman at all, but as

---

[75] Office of Pesticide Programs, EPA, *Acetochlor: Desk Statement, March 11, 1994* www.epa.gov/oppefd1/aceto/index.

he looks into JoAn's eyes, he sees the same haunted look he has come to know in himself.

Many weeks later, after being diagnosed with untreatable cancer, they had been in bed asleep one night when all at once Jim heard a blood curdling scream, the source of which was only inches from his ear. This was like something he had never experienced before, except possibly at a horror flick. But this was no horror film. This was very real. This was his lover in unbearable pain.

For JoAn the cancer was as relentless as the probable causes; and as relentless as the passage of time. In this case, however, the causes of cancer team up in a most potent way. Time waits for no one and nothing. Neither does cancer. Once the carcinogens enter the body, there is no waiting around. Oh, it may take years before the cancer begins to grow and spread, but the cancer is not going to disappear just because measures are now being taken to rid or reduce the environment of those same carcinogenic elements.

There is little comfort for JoAn's family today that:

- DDT was banned in 1972, or that
- Cyanazine was banned in 2002.

Nor, is there any comfort for Jim that in 1992, the very year the "Attack on JoAn" began, Lewis Regenstein, a Pulitzer nominee, was preparing the public with the warning:

Over two decades after being largely 'banned' in the United States, DDT is still killing Americans, most recently being implicated in the CURRENT EPIDEMIC OF BREAST CANCER....[76]

It would be of even less comfort to read the conclusion drawn four-years before JoAn's death by Cook & Dresser that breast cancer "is uncommon in women under the age of 35.[77] In fact, Jim would bitterly note that for once JoAn beat the odds!

Already by 1992 the carcinogens present in Donna Jo's body, JoAn's, Susan's, and Sandra's had picked up speed. Time was running out for each one of them – and countless others in not just Fremont County, Iowa, but for millions throughout the world. As

---

[76] Regenstein, 338; emphasis added.
[77] Alan R. Cook and Peter D. Dresser, eds., <u>Cancer Sourcebook for Women</u> (Detroit: Omnigraphics, Inc., 19960, 25

Watts & Williamson rightly relate in their book <u>Replacing Chemicals with Biology</u>.[78]

> *Pesticides have been poisoning farm workers, their families and communities for over 60 years. Yet there is still no accurate estimate of the degree of human suffering from exposure to pesticides. The most authoritative study available today is one published in the <u>World Health Statistics Quarterly</u> in 1990, using data derived in the 1980 – nearly 30 years ago. This study estimated that there were possibly one million of cases so serious unintentional pesticide poisonings each year, and an additional two million cases of people hospitalized for suicide attempts with pesticides. The author noted that this necessarily reflected only a fraction of the real problem and estimated that there could be as many as 25 million agricultural workers in the developing world suffering from occupational pesticide poisoning each year, though most incidents are not recorded, and most patients do not seek medical attention. A more recent surveillance in Central America indicated a 98 percent rate of underreporting of pesticide poisonings, with a regional estimate of 400,000 poisonings per year, 76 percent of the incidents being work related.*

---

[78] Watts & Williamson, 17-18, citing J. Jeyaratnam 1990, "Acute Pesticide Poisoning: A Major Global Health Problem," <u>World Health Stat Q 43 (3): 139-144,</u> et al studies.

Chapter Four

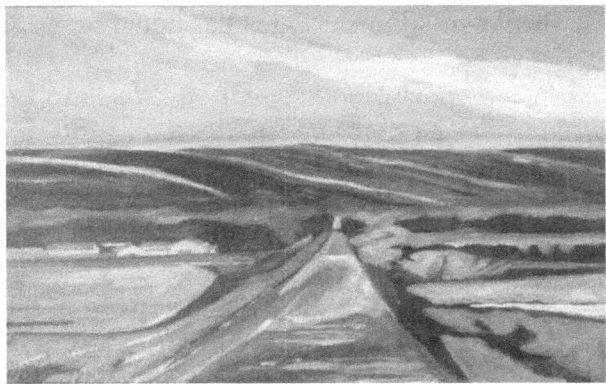

Homeward

Multiplicity of Causes: How Many Ways to Die?

So far, the discussion here has centered mainly on rural locations or, at most rural towns. However, even cities are not immune from being victimized by this form of chemical warfare. If pesticides invade ground water, underlying aquifers will be infected as well. The USGS noted in 1998, for example, that the Ashland well-field in Nebraska which "provides almost all of the water for the city of Lincoln[79]…" was comparable in levels of detected atrazine to the highest samples, rates "as high as 20mg/L."[80] In fact, the USGS also reported "the Platte River alluvial scored among the highest 25 percent nationally for percent detection of pesticides."[81]

Furthermore, this is also true for any area relying upon relatively shallow water tables for drinking water supplies. As the Iowa Department of Natural Resources cites: "The greatest proportions of contaminated wells occur … (where) nearly 75% of

---

[79] NOTE: Lincoln's estimated population in 2017 was 284,736, the second largest city in Nebraska); see *World Population Review* at: www.worldpopulationreview.com/us-cities/lincoln-population.

[80] 20 mg/L = 20 milligrams of atrazine per liter of water.

[81] USGS, Water Quality in the Central Nebraska Basin, 4, 6.

wells are <100 feet deep..."[82] Nearly all wells in the Fremont County area are shallow wells with 50 feet being the most common. As the President's Cancer Panel has noted"

An analysis of more than two million drinking water test results acquired from 42 state water offices found 260 contaminants in tap water. Of these, 141 contaminants have no safety standards.

Forty (40)of the unregulated contaminants were detected in tap water consumed by at least one million people.[83]

It is not just the pesticides that come at us from the many sources already noted here. In 1996, John Wargo was able to claim that as far as the then available pesticides were concerned "few of their metabolites and none of their 1600 inert ingredients have been examined for their health effects and still remain unregulated as possible food contaminants."[84] To make matters worse, modern medical science has little-to-no knowledge of how the effects of even low pesticide levels weigh upon human health, to say nothing about the interaction of combinations of them all, their metabolites and the inert components.[85] Worse yet, the President's Cancer Panel warns us that:

Tens of thousands more chemicals and other substances are in us that never have been evaluated and whose carcinogenicity unknown.[86] And: In the U.S., about 42 billion pounds of chemicals are produced or imported daily. Many of these chemicals are used in massive quantities exceeding one million tons per year.[87]

---

[82] Iowa Department of Natural Resources, Geological Survey Bureau. The Iowa State-Wide Rural Well-Water Survey: Water-Quality Data: Initial Analysis (Abstract), September 19, 1990. www.igsb.uuiowa.edu/gsbpubs/abstracts/TIS-19.

[83] PCP 2010, 54; citing Environmental Working Group, A national assessment of tap water quality, (September 18, 20098) www.ewg.org/tapwater/findings.php.

[84] Wargo, 7.

[85] Iowa Association of Naturalists, Iowa Agricultural Practices & the Environment, Iowa Environmental Issues Series (September 1998), 9.

[86] PCP 2010, 29.

[87] Ibid, 16; citing National Pollution Prevention and Toxics Advisory Committee, Broader Issues Working Group, Initial Thought Starter: How can EPA more efficiently identify potential risks and facilitate risk reduction decisions for non-

We spread it on our lawns and golf courses as well.[88] In fact the EPA has determined that 91% of American households use pesticides while another report found that homeowners use more pesticides per acre than do agricultural users.[89] The USGS reported in 2001:

Herbicides are widespread in surface water (detected in 99% of urban stream samples)and ground water (detected in 50% of sampled wells). Most common are those applied to lawns, golf courses and road rights-of-ways, such as atrazine, simazine, and prometon.[90]

Chemigation

Rural communities are exposed to chemical drift from nearby farmland, either through the air via aerial spraying, or by inhaling the mists from chemigation – the mixing of pesticides with the center pivot's spray irrigation of crops.[91] The resulting mist from chemigation can be carried into towns, as well as across the pastures to farmsteads.

Unwell Wells

A rural community's otherwise safe water supply may become infected by pesticides first seeping into "abandoned or poorly constructed (nearby farm) wells… (I)f the well is not protected properly or if the pipes or tiles are old and cracked, the pesticides may contaminate the well and reach the groundwater."[92] This very

---

HPV chemicals? (Nov 6, 2005, cited July 17, 2009) www.epa.gov/oppt/npptac/pubs/finaldraftnonhpvpaper051006.PDF.

[88] Office of Pesticide Programs, EPA (Aug '99), 2. **NOTE:** to be cited hereafter as OPP, EPA, Aug '99.

[89] Iowa Association of Naturalists, Iowa Water Pollution, Iowa Environmental Issues Series, September 1998, 11 (to be cited hereafter as Iowa Water Pollution).

[90] USGS, Selected Findings and Current Perspectives on Urban and Agricultural Water Quality by the National Water-Quality Assessment Program, (USGS, April 2001; FS-047-01. **NOTE:** To be cited hereafter as "Selected Findings."

[91] Strange, 289.

[92] Iowa Water Pollution, 8.

common problem makes a mockery of Robert Frost's nostalgic poem about the restorative powers of water:

Directive[93]
Back out of all this too much for us,
Back in a time made simple by the loss
Of detail, burned, dissolved, and broken off
Like a graveyard marble sculpture in the weather,
There is a house that is no more a house
Upon a farm that is no more a farm
And a town that is no more a town…

Your destination and your destiny's
A brook that was the water of the house,
Cold as a spring as yet so near its source.

Here are your waters and your watering place.
Drink and be whole again beyond confusion.
                    (Robert Frost)

Multiple Chemical Exposure & Sensitivities

Let us count the ways the four women recounted here so far could have been exposed to pesticides:
- Ingesting their mother's milk,
- Eating pesticide-laden baby food,
- Drinking from the shallow wells at home and at school,
- Breathing-in the contaminated air from aerial spraying or chemigation, or both,
- Inhaling the mix of pesticides in the water used for bathing and showering,[94]

---

[93] Joel Conarroe, ed., Six American Poets (NY: Random House, 1991), 221-223.
[94] In 1984 a Rockford, Illinois, electroplating company had polluted 150 private wells and a municipal well. Subsequent monitoring of the families affected resulted in the conclusion that chemical levels in their carefully monitored blood "correlated with air levels more than with water contaminant levels, and air levels correlated with "**length of shower run times.**" [From: Steingraber #1, citing J.E. Keller and S.W. Metcalf, "Exposure Study of Volatile Organic Compounds in

- Eating polluted food, including fish from the river,[95]
- Swimming in a community pool "purified' and "sanitized" with the pesticide simazine,[96]
- Wearing their DDT-based dry-cleaned clothes,
- Breathing-in DDT at home, at work, or while seated in a commercial airline,
- Being exposed to multiple combinations of the above,
- Unknowingly being open to multiple combinations of pesticides and their multiple metabolites, or multiple combinations of the above,
- Daily exposures to all-of-the-above, and perhaps even more.

While recognizing there are many agents that can potentially cause cancer, such as nuclear fallout, nuclear waste, and nuclear radiation release, certain antihistamines and antidepressants,[97] smoking and urban air pollution, the focus here is on pesticides. How many such exposures does it take to activate cancer cells? No one knows. The question appears to have been avoided by medical science. It is, admittedly, a very complex question. The empirical challenges are enormous. So too would be the cost of researching the dynamics and effects of multiple chemical exposures. The much heralded and important Long Island Breast Cancer Study Project (LIBCSP), begun in 1993 and spending more than $19,000,000 as of 2000, fails, according to Dr. Janette Sherman, in 'NOT (emphasis added) addressing the additive and synergistic effects from exposure to multiple chemicals and multiple radiation emissions."[98]

Southeast Rockford," Epidemiological Report Series 91:3 (Springfield, ILL: IDPH, 1991]. Emphasis added.

[95] Streams where row cops dominate the drainage basin had large concentrations of nutrients (nitrates) and pesticides in the water, **the largest residues of pesticides in fish tissues, and degraded fish communities**." [From: Water Quality in the Central Nebraska Basin, 2), Emphasis added.

[96] "In 1994, the EPA removed the swimming pool use from all simazine labels due to the Agency's concerns over the risks to people from exposure to simazine residues in swimming pool water." [OPP, EPA (Aug '99), 2].

[97] Janette Sherman, Life's Delicate Balance: Causes and Prevention of Breast Cancer (NY: Taylor & Francis, 2000), 21-24.

[98] Ibid, 178.

In a USGS 1999 report it was noted that:

Long-term exposures to low-level mixtures of pesticide compounds, punctuated with seasonal pulses of higher concentrations is the most common pattern of exposure, but the effects of this pattern are not yet well understood.[99]

However, it is well understood that childhood exposure to pesticides is riskier than for adults due to the more rapid rate of cell division in children than for adults. As the American Academy of Pediatrics (AAP) states it, "Children encounter pesticides every day and are uniquely vulnerable to their toxicity."[100]

The USGS warns in its 2001 report that while:

Concentrations of pesticides are low and below drinking water standards...the risk to humans and the environment from present-day levels of contaminant exposure remains unclear. For example, current standards and guidelines do not yet account for exposure to mixtures, and many pesticides and their breakdown products do not have standards or guidelines.[101]

Some work, however, has been done on what is known as Multiple Chemical Exposure (MCE) and is strongly suggestive of how it was that the women chronicled herein contracted the lethal disease that took their lives. Multiple Chemical Sensitivity (MCS),

...is a phenomenon whereby individuals report an increased sensitivity to chemicals in the environment and attribute their sensitivities to prior chemical exposure.[102]

---

[99] USGS Survey, 1999, <u>The Quality of Our Nations Waters – Nutrients and Pesticides</u>, (USGS Circular 1225).

[100] American Academy of Pediatrics, "AAP Makes Recommendations to Reduce Children's Exposure to Pesticides," November 26, 2012 www.aap.org/en-us/about-the-aap/aap-press-room.

[101] USGS, "Selected Findings."

[102] Dr. Barbara A. Sorg, "Multiple Chemical Sensitivities," <u>Agrichemical and Environmental News</u>, March 1999, Issue N, 155 (Cooperative Extension, Washington State University; originally accessed. But no longer available at: www.tricity.wsu.edu/aenews/Mar99AENews; now available at www.aenews.wsu.edu (accessed February 2, 2016).

MCS is the symptoms people experience due to concentrated exposures from such events a pesticide factory chemical spills, as well as those symptoms associated with the Persian Gulf War Syndrome. Common MCS symptoms include, extreme fatigue, headaches, gastrointestinal disorders, muscle and joint pains, depression, memory and concentration difficulties, irritability and mood swings, dizziness, anxiety, formation of ovarian cysts, and upper respiratory irritations.[103] MCS is a two-phased process.

First, the *Initiation Phase:*
...thought to be the stage during which either repeated exposure to chemicals, a high-level chemical exposure (such as that occurring during a chemical spill), or other stressful life events initiate the process of later sensitivity to chemicals.[104]

For those affected by MCS due to such experiences, the initiation phase is quick, immediate, and sometimes absolutely harrowing. For the Donna Jo's the initiation phase may be gradual and un-observed over a very longtime.

Second, the *Elicitation Phase, or Triggering,* is when MCS-prone individuals:

...report exquisite sensitivity to odors and feelings of illness from chemical exposures encountered at home and workplace.[105]

The women storied here all began experiencing almost all of the MCS symptoms, in most cases, years before a diagnosis of cancer was handed to them. Mike recalls that as many as ten years prior to Donna Jo's diagnosis there were episodes when this normally dynamic, upbeat, energetic woman who never knew illness would

---

[103] Ibid.

[104] Ibid.

[105] Ibid. NOTE, also, that MCS is similar to the concept of Chronic Toxicity – the *toxic effects (e.g., cancer) usually occurring weeks, months, or years after exposure to a toxic agent or as a result of long-term, low-level exposure.* (FROM: "The Science and Politics of Pesticides," by C.F. Wilkinson in Silent Spring Revisited, Gino G. Marco, ed, [Washington: American Chemical Society, 1987, 44].

experience nausea or would become surprisingly moody, depressed and totally devoid of enough energy to get out of her chair.

The parallel between MCE/MCS and the probable chemical causes of cancer seem much too suggestive to be ignored any longer, especially when we note that:

> *Approximately four times more women are affected than men are and the average onset (i.e., elicitation/triggering) is in the fourth decade.*[106]

For every one of these Iowa women their cancer symptoms first appeared in the fourth decade of their lives.

However, research on MCE is slow due to its complexity and difficulty in executing traditional empirical research techniques, such as reliable double-blind cohort studies, and having to rely on anecdotal data. The latter is generally viewed by medical science as unreliable. It has been too easy and too convenient to dismiss patients' narratives as flights of the imagination, health-related environmental coincidences, or episodes of hypochondria.

Barbara Sorg, Professor, Department of Veterinary and Comparative Anatomy, Pharmacology, and Physiology at Washington State University, implores medical science to take off its blinders and accept the fact that:

> *The symptoms experienced by MCS patients are real. Our lack of understanding should not provide a rationale to dismiss symptoms purely as part of a (scientific or medical) belief system. Instead, the absence of knowledge should provide impetus to initiate rigorous, scientific studies to help verify or refute claims that chemical exposures initiate/trigger MCS illness.*[107]

Grace Ziem, M.D., who works in the field of Occupational and Environmental Medicine (OEM), has no hesitation in observing that:

---

[106] Sorg.
[107] Ibid.

MCS often develops after repeated symptomatic exposure to petrochemicals including *exposure to pesticides....[108]*

If the impact upon individual or a community's health cannot possibly gain proper recognition as an actionable issue, then perhaps the issue needs to be reframed. Instead of an appeal as a public health issue, an appeal that oftentimes is interpreted as an altruistic issue, perhaps the substantive issue itself needs to be defined in terms a capitalist economy and a capitalist political system can better understand. Note, for example, the findings of such experts as the then Deputy State Epidemiologist of New Mexico. In 1998, Dr. Ron Voorhees "estimated…that the State may be losing 15 million dollars a year in tax revenues due to decreased earning capacity of those with MCS."[109]

Furthermore, a group of leading endocrinologists, in early 2015,

Concluded with 99% certainty that environmental exposure to hormone disrupting chemicals causes health problems. They estimate that this costs the European Union Health care system about $175 billion a year.[110]

The President's Cancer Panel states the case well:

Scientific evidence on individual and multiple environmental exposure effects on disease initiation and outcomes and consequent health system and societal costs are not being adequately integrated into national policy decisions and strategies for disease prevention, health care access, and health system reform.[111]

---

[108] Grace Ziem, "Understanding Patients with Multiple Chemical Sensitivity," Letter to the Editor, <u>American Family Physician</u>; www.aafp.org/afp/990415ap/letters.

[109] Ann McCampbell, M.D., "Multiple Chemical Sensitivities Under Siege." www.getipm.com/personal/mcs-campbell.

[110] Valerie Brown and Elizabeth Grossman, "Why the United States Leaves Deadly Chemicals on the Market," <u>In These Times</u> (November 2, 2015), 19 pp. www.inthesetimes.magazine.com Accessed November 28, 2015).

[111] PCP 2010, vii.

Chapter Five

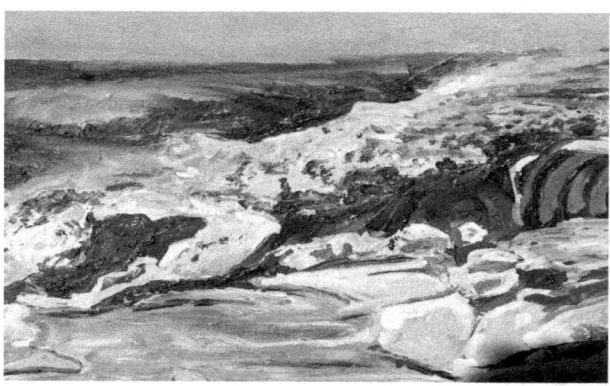

Run-off Ditch

Ambiguities of Environmental Monitoring

As just noted, there is hardly unanimity in medical science regarding MCE and MCS, dynamics, causes or consequences – or even it it is worth studying. Equally, there is little agreement about the impact of exposure to low levels of pesticides on human health.[112] In fact there appears to be about as much agreement among medical researchers on these issues as there is in a book discussion group I belonged to whenever we discussed any author's intent or even if the book was worth reading. Much seems to depend upon the reader's worldview and values. Much of the dissonance in medical science lies with the ambiguities of cause and effect, the ambiguities of measurement monitoring, as well as the scientist's worldview and values.

Reading some of the literature, however, would lead one to believe that ambiguity has long since been replaced with precision and certainty. Listen to just one example:

...45 percent of the shallow wells sampled in the Platte Valley and more than 25 percent of the shallow wells in the Glaciated Area exceed the USEPA's MCL (Maximum Contaminant Level) of 10milligrams per liter (mg/L)...Median nitrate

---

[112] Iowa Water Pollution, 11.

concentrations in areas with shallow depths to ground water and undergoing intensely irrigated cropland that is dominated by corn production…were more than twice the MVL of 10 mg/L for drinking water.[113]

Initially, one would have the impression that the scientific tools are well developed, the definitions clear, but that is hardly the case. Sandra Steingraber, who is both a scientist and a women's health advocate, states the problem well:

*For many chemicals, two numbers exist: the enforceable Maximum and the health-based maximum contaminant-level goals, officially defined as a 'non-enforceable concentration of a drinking water contaminant that is protective of adverse human health effects and allows an adequate margin of safety. The enforceable values for the carcinogens, benzene, vinyl chloride, and trichloroethylene…have been set at 5, 2, and 5 parts per billion, respectively. Their maximum-contaminant-level goals, however are all zero…**It ignores exposures to combinations of chemicals that may act in concert.**[114]*

The latter point, of course, takes us back to a concern related to the reality for many people with MCS.

From here-on let us refer to the enforceable maximum contaminant level goal (EMCLG) as the *enforceable limit* and the health-based maximum contaminant level goal (HBMCLG) as the *health-based goal.* The EMCLGs are based on generalizations, averages and medians; that is, statistics that relate to the general population and to the environment. Clearly, they can be nothing but goals. We have, perhaps to use the analogy from the game of football, a long-since squandering of opportunities to cross the goal line of complete eradication, due to a whole series of hideous plays, neglectful coaching, and even some of the players throwing the game for profit. More on that later. The focus now is the role of neglect.

---

[113] "Major Issues and Findings – Nitrate Content in Water is Related to Agricultural Land Management," USGS, <u>Water Quality in the Central Nebraska Basins</u>, 1-2.
[114] Steingraber #1, 194; emphasis added.

It would seem, in terms of human health and consequences for human suffering, the governmental insistence of pursuing *enforceable limits* as a policy goal compromises public health. In effect, it claims that some unknown numbers of compromised health is perfectly fine. Of course, one must acknowledge that the *enforceable limit* concept is better than doing nothing. On the other hand, a *health-based goal*, which would permit no compromise, by setting a zero-tolerance level, would prevent countless numbers of people falling between the cracks of statistical averages and early death.

Even after the Rural Water Treatment Act became law, "small water suppliers in nearly every state have been completely exempt from controlling levels of chlorination byproducts and from testing for CBPs.[115] Given EPA's definition of "small supplier" (those serving less than 10,000 people), we find that between 1996 and 2001, alone, 1000 such public water systems reported at least one uninterrupted 12 month period where the toxic level exceeded standards that were scheduled to go into effect in2002. That means at least 5600 bladder cancer cases annually[116] were likely to have been caused in part by neglect. As Robert Wayland, former director of the Office of Wetlands, Oceans and Watersheds, observes:

You don't find what you don't look for.[117]

Contamination Case # 1:
Former Pesticide Plant, Shenandoah, Iowa

A pesticide plant operated in Shenandoah, Iowa, from 1961 to 1973, when a fire destroyed the chemical warehouse, leaving only an office building. In 1974, a seed company purchased the building. The new

---

[115] Consider the Source: Farm runoff; chlorination byproducts, and human health (Washington, DC: Environmental Working Group and U.S. Public Interest Research Group, Oct 2001, 27).

[116] Ibid. The 5600 bladder cancer cases are extrapolated from the EPA's estimate that 7000 such cases would have occurred annually across the 1258 public water supplies reporting the reporting the same toxic excess as cited for small suppliers.

[117] "Lack of Water Quality Standards for Pesticides," Beyond Pesticides Daily News Archive, March 26, 2002.
www.beyondpesticides.org/NEWS/daily_news_archives/03_26_02.html.

owner, knowing the site's history, buttressed by input from former employees of the pesticide plant, finally, after nearly 14 years, consented to a series of site environmental assessments. These evaluations were conducted in 1988, 1993, 1994, 1995 and 1998.

`The site was assessed for pesticide exposure risk to the population, and a "risk-based" *Enforceable Limit* known as a "Reasonable Maximum Exposure" (RME) was established by the assessing agency. The RME (to be referred to here-in as *Reasonable Exposure*) in this case the "highest exposure that is reasonably expected to occur at the site. *Reasonable Exposure* is a high-end estimate (above the 90th percentile) of exposure to a population."[118]

There will be no argument here whether Maximum Contaminant Levels (MCLs) need to be set. Clearly, they must. In an ideal world, perhaps, we would have one MCL and one MCL only – a *Health-Based Goal.* In other words, all MCLs for all chemicals and toxic substances in all geographic situations related to all potentially affected populations would be set at zero. Otherwise, we would never cross the goal line. If getting to the 10-yard line is always considered "good enough," the "game" will always be forfeited from the beginning.

The standards of monitoring and measurement are far too ambiguous as they related to the goal of public health and safety. The general standards neglect the individual.

The *Reasonable Exposure* noted above totally ignores the question of Multiple Chemical Exposure and/or Multiple Chemical Sensitivity for the one person nearby, the few people nearby, or the dozens and hundreds whose lives may be endangered. Using the logic of the operative RME in the case of the former pesticide plant in Shenandoah, and allowing that 10% of the population could be detrimentally affected leads to the following conclusion:

With a population of 5572 people in 1990, there is a potential that 557 folks would suffer detrimental effects from residual pesticide contamination. Under the RME, this is statistically and (apparently) medically, politically, administratively, morally, and ethically acceptable. Acceptable to whom? The 557 citizens of Shenandoah and their loved ones? No. It is acceptable ONLY to the policy makers. Clearly, the limits of acceptability need to be altered

---

[118] Health Consultation, See "Discussion."

with prejudice in favor of the public good, and away from corporate profit.

Would these same decision-makers come to the same decisions if their own health and safety were involved? The answer, perhaps, lies within an incident described by Michael Pollan:

A potato farmer in Idaho, Danny Forsythe, who utilizes massive amounts of Monsanto chemicals to raise his crops, explains to Pollan:

> *I like to eat organic food, and in fact I grow a lot of it at the house. The vegetables we buy at the market we just wash and wash and wash. I'm not sure I should be saying this, but I always plant a small area of potatoes without any chemicals. By the end of the season, my field of potatoes are fine to eat, but any potatoes I pulled today are probably still full of systemics. I don't eat them.*[119]

Furthermore, what are the implications for the unborn child who could have been one of the 10th percentile potentially affected at a critical moment of formation in the mother's womb? We wonder at the implications for the adolescent girl and all such girls whose breasts were beginning to form at a time when they could have been exposed to any one or more of the following pesticides detected "between the south site boundary and the nearest residence": Aldrin, Dieldrin, DDE, DDT, Gamma Chlordane, and Methoxychlor.[120]

What are the implications for a woman of any age nearby whose multiple chemical sensitive body was "just waiting" for the triggering action of one more exposure – an exposure that could set off the growth of cancer-bearing tumors? The implications for Helen and her husband Ben, both of whom worked at the old pesticide plant (and lived no more than a few blocks from the south site boundary) seem quite clear.

****

August 1999
HELEN (1918-2000) was dying of ovarian cancer. It was a hot day in August when I first met her. She was still a very independent person, living by herself. Her only child, Mitzie, checked in on

---

[119] Michael Pollan, The Botany of Desire: A Plant's – Eye View of the World (Random House, 2001, 223).
[120] Health Consultation, See "Site Inspection 1993."

Helen routinely early in the morning, at noon, right after work, and later in the evening – seven days a week of vigilant care giving.

My knock on the door evokes an order from within the house to "Come In!" And so it was that I found this bright 82 year-old woman, blighted by the cancer that was slowly diminishing her life, sitting in a recliner, wrapped in a blanket, all windows closed and AC shut off. While I am soon sweltering, Helen complains of being "so cold."

As we talk, the conversation shifts from her illness to her family, and to her deceased husband, Ben. She claims he died of prostate cancer six years before. I am slowly struck by something very different about this woman. She has NOT raised the "why" and "how" questions others have uttered. Helen has the answers.

"Ben worked his whole life at the old pesticide plant here in Shenandoah. I worked there, as well. Never knew anyone who ever worked there to NOT have cancer, and eventually die of it, like I'm fixin' to do!"

While the cleanup of the former pesticide plant, as ordered by the USEPA, could prevent future compromises to public health arising from this site, it makes no difference now to Helen and Ben. They are both dead.

One might argue, reasonably and accurately, that perfection in measurement and monitoring is an elusive goal. Surely it is. However, the standards of measurement touted by the USEPA, the Office of Pesticide Programs, and the Agency for Toxic Substances and Disease Registry, turn out to be deceptively ambiguous, lax and permissive. For example, as of 1996 *Enforceable Limits* had been set for only 84 contaminants. The President's Cancer Panel claims that as of 2009 the U.S. National toxicology Program's (NTP) Report on Carcinogens "lists 246 agents as known carcinogens or substances 'reasonably anticipated to be human carcinogens.'"[121]

When it comes to monitoring water contamination, assessments are often based on annual averages of four quarterly measurements. In these cases, a community's drinking water standard would be violated in a given year when the yearly mean

---

[121] PCP 2010, p.29. citing NTP Program Report on Carcinogens, 11th ed. Research Triangle Park (NC): National Institute for Environmental Health Sciences, 2005. http://nieha.nih.gov.

concentration of a particular contaminant might be found in excess of the *Enforceable Limits.*[122]

What are the implications for people in those communities where the yearly mean average is .01 below the *Enforceable Limit,* but where spring run-off of pesticides from cropland spurs an occasional daily exceedingly high level of contamination? The yearly mean may satisfy the *Enforceable Limit* standard, but what are the implications for the children's growing bodies as they consume daily doses of atrazine? What are the implications for the chemically sensitive folks? Is it the dose of cyanazine residue in the well water on a given day that triggers cancer in one's prostate?

A common standard of measurement in the monitoring of surface or ground water contaminant levels is 10 milligrams per liter (10mg/L). It certainly was of no comfort for people in Central Nebraska to hear from the USGS in 1998 that even while "most stringent fertilizer-management guidelines" had been followed since 1986, "nearly 25 percent of the wells in the area continued to exceed 20 mg/L in 1994...."[123] Keep in mind that the 20mg+/L condition/violation represented at least twice the 10mg/L level considered to be safe for human consumption.

What are the implications for human beings exposed to water infused with atrazine at a rate 30% below what USEPA considers safe? We know what that same level of atrazine-tainted water does to frogs. It produces hermaphroditism.[124]

What are the implications for those women who work in the fields harvesting lettuce in the Salinas Valley of California? We know the answer to that one: their children are born with brain abnormalities due to their mothers' exposure to pesticides such as the chemical chlorpyrifos. Plus, we know those mothers, the

---

[122] Steingraber #1, 195.

[123] Water Quality in the Central Nebraska Basins 1995, 4.

[124] Rachel Aviv, "A Valuable Reputation: After Tyrone Hayes said that a chemical was harmful, its maker pursued him." (The New Yorker, February 10, 2014); www.newyorker.com/magazine/2014/02/10/a-valuable-reputation. Accessed February 11, 2015. [See Chapter 8 for full discussion of Dr. Tyrone Hayes's ordeals for disclosing the truth].

CHAMACOS mothers, "harbored higher levels of pesticide metabolites than most Americans."[125]

However, we do not have a clear idea what the implications are for the 25% of American pregnant women who "harbored pesticide concentrations <u>higher than the median levels measured in the CHAMACOS mothers.</u>"[126]

What are the implications for the family whose drinking water ranked somewhere among the other 75% of wells that weighed in with a reading of 9.9md/L and was, therefore considered safe; to say nothing about the murky issue of the effect of combinations of chemicals?

Dr. Bruce Lanphear, a public health physician and professor of Health Sciences at Simon Fraser University in British Columbia, Canada, provides a sobering answer to all the implication questions above:

"THERE IS NO SAFE LEVEL OF EXPOSURE."[127]

Contamination Case # 2:
Bruno, Nebraska

Now, let us consider the event in Bruno,[128] Nebraska, where people in the community raised their concerns about the local grain storage facility as a possible contaminant of the public water supply.[129] The community was aroused about:

---

[125] Susan Freunkel, "Pesticides and the Young Brain," <u>The Nation</u>) (March 31, 2014), 12-22. CHAMACOS: Center for the Health Assessment of Mothers and Children of Salinas. NOTE: Chamacos is Mexican slang for "little kids" (p.14).

[126] Ibid, 18 (emphasis added).

[127] Dr. Bruce Lanphear, "Little things matter: the impact of toxins on the developing brain," <u>www.youtube.com/Watch?v=E6KomAb2BW</u> ; and "Pesticides at even low levels harmful to children," (<u>The Hindu</u>, September 7, 2015. <u>www.thehindu.com/news/national/kerala/pesticides-at-low-levels-impact-children</u>, Accessed October 8, 2015.

[128] Bruno, Nebraska, named in honor of the Czech city of Brno.

[129] <u>Public Health Assessment: Bruno Coop & Associated Properties, Bruno, Butler County, Nebraska, 1994</u>. <u>www.atsdr.cdc.gov/HAC/PHA/bruno</u> (to be cited herein after as <u>Public Health Assessment: Bruno</u>).

- *Cancerous and non-cancerous health effects resulting from exposure to contaminants found in the old water supply.*
- *The relationship between carbon tetrachloride and development of hepatitis.*
- *The health effects from eating crops, which have been irrigated with the contaminated water.*[130]

Following extensive study of the situation in Bruno, the Agency for Toxic Substances and Disease Registry (ATSDR, a federal agency under the Center for Disease Control) concluded there was "No apparent public health hazard." Yet, in the paragraph immediately preceding this conclusion we find it said that:

- *Use of carbon tetrachloride (CC14), 1,2-dichloroethane, and chloroform at the grain facility appears to be the dominant source of chemicals found in groundwater and in soil gas.*
- *People were likely exposed to contaminants in the water supply...by ingesting the contaminated water or by breathing in or direct skin contact with chemicals while engaging in various activities such as showering.*

No apparent public health hazard? Let us carefully examine this report:

The Bruno co-op property was originally owned and operated by the C&NW Railway Company. From 1947 to the 1960's, the US Department of Agriculture leased it as a federal grain storage facility. In the mid-1960's, the Bruno Coop purchased some of the property, but the Agrico Chemical Company, also at one time, leased a portion of the land for use in "storing, blending and distributing anhydrous ammonia and related products."[131]

The ATSDR examiners were told that:

---

[130] Ibid, see "Summary."
[131] Ibid. see "Background."

- *The chemicals (*noted above*) were banned for fumigant use (by the Bruno Coop) in the mid-1980s, and the USDA stopped using them in the mid-1960s.*
- *Neither fumigants nor those chemicals have been used on the property for at least the past two years – the manager's term of service.*
- *All the inhabited residences in Bruno are connected to the public water supply but have wells that are used to water lawns.*
- *A well survey had not been conducted for the area.[132]*

ATSDR then sampled ground water for the public wells and one private well, finding that "contaminants have been released into the groundwater, soil, and air." The agency then plugged into their formulary the *Cancer Risk Evaluation Guide (CREG)* (to be referred to herein as *(Cancer Risk Guide)*. The Guide is an "estimated comparison of concentrations for specific chemicals based on an excess cancer rate of one in a million persons…" The ATSDR goes on to note that water samples taken from the two old public wells and from water taps in homes between 1984 and 1989 indicated "contaminants attributed to grain storage chemical treatment activities were found at levels that exceed ATSDR's comparison values for drinking water use for Cc14, chloroform, and DCA.[133]

Then, the blockbuster:

Analyses suggest there are completed pathways associated with groundwater and pesticide uses. Affected populations include residents and grain storage workers.

The ATSDR report immediately follows up by boldly stating seven conclusions:
- The three contaminants noted before were present in the two old public wells, albeit "typically at low

---

[132] Ibid.
[133] Ibid. see "Environmental Contamination and Other Hazards."

61

concentrations...Therefore within some part of the time between the 1940s and 1990. Residents, workers, and visitors were exposed to those chemicals principally through ingestion and inhalation (showering and cooking). Exposure also occurred through skin contact."

- "Spraying, pouring, or dumping fumigant chemicals...is believed to have resulted in exposure to persons that applied the chemicals through inhalation, skin contact, and incidental ingestion. ATSDR was told that fumigators were 'overcome' when using chemicals at storage units owned by a former operator."

- "Residents, workers, and visitors in the community are being exposed intermittently – now and possibly in the future – to **low levels of chlorination by-product chemicals.**[134] This exposure pathway is unrelated to releases at the site."

- "ATSDR believes private well use is the most important of the potential exposure pathways. Available data are not sufficient to evaluate the pathway."

- "Soil gas might enter and accumulate in residences (principally those with basements)... Information is not available to adequately evaluate the pathway."

- "Chemicals poured into rodent holes, and possibly those used excessively to fumigate grain, would have contaminated some of the subsurface soils...Thus any workers – past, present, and future – that engage in excavation might be exposed to residual levels of those chemicals through skin contact, inhalation, and incidental ingestion. Data are not available to evaluate that potential exposure."

- Persons that use private Wells for irrigation (for example, lawns, crops), potentially are exposed – past, present, future –principally through skin contact...Analytical data are not available to evaluate that potential exposure."[135]

Repeating the foregoing litany:

---

[134] Emphasis added.
[135] Ibid. see "Pathways Analyses.

- Available data are not sufficient to evaluate the pathway.
- Information is not available to adequately evaluate the pathway.
- Data are not available to evaluate that potential exposure.
- Analytical data are not available to evaluate that potential exposure.

While often citing the lack of conclusive studies and/or any data linking, for example, exposure to CC14 with cancer, the report goes on to conclude that:

1. There is **"no apparent public health hazard currently"** and
2. The site is classified as an **"indeterminate public health hazard for past exposures."**[136]

Yes, the data were not available. But while the Bruno study was being done, and while the expense of the study was being incurred, and whole people's lives are at stake, why was the next step not taken? To conclude that there is an indefinite current risk, and to do no more, seems to be an injustice to the residents of Bruno.

Much of the grist for the conclusions of **no apparent current risk** and **indefinite past risk** appears to come from the reluctance to rely on, or take seriously, the scientifically "suspect" anecdotal data. While citing the stories shared with the ATSDR regarding fumigators being "overcome" by the chemical, the ATSDR investigators simply note that:

Due to lack of information including the concentration of chemical components within the fumigants, frequency of fumigation, and specific type of adverse effect(s)...ATSDR is unable to quantitatively or qualitatively evaluate these exposures.[137]

But did they try? Was it even considered? Was any thought ever given to the possibility of tracking down the employees who had been "overcome" and to ask them the pertinent questions? They would have accurate knowledge of the concentrations of chemicals

---

136 Ibid. see "Conclusions."
137 Ibid. see "Public Health Implications."

they were using, the frequency of fumigation, and the frequency of being "overcome," to say nothing about the adverse effects they experienced. Sadly, this extension of the "Public Health assessment did not happen.

*****

SHELLEY (1955-2000)[138] was born and raised in a house adjacent to the Bruno Grain Elevator. Try telling Shelley's family there is an "indeterminant public health hazard for past exposures" in Bruno. They are quite aware of the consequences of living next to the Agrico Chemical Company and the Bruno Coop-, as well as having lived in a community surrounded by cornfields irrigated and fumigated by way of chemigation.

Shelley lived the first 18 years of her life in one of the two homes currently vacant and unconnected to the public water supply at the time of the ATSDR study of the Coop site. Her father worked at the Agrico facility and later at the Coop. When she was about 8 years-old, Agrico began operating across the street from her home. There was always good loose and easily dug dirt that Shelley and her friends could carry off in their buckets for the big sandbox her father had built for her in the side yard. The "Dirt Brigade" would steal across the street at night and quickly, deftly fill their buckets and scurry back. Shelley and her friends loved playing in the dirt that 34 years later would be declared contaminated soil, which most likely was freshly contaminated at the time of the children's play.

The family initially thought their water supply was okay, but they came to know differently. When relatives from out-of-town visited, Shelley's parents were often gently reminded that their water was NOT okay. There was just a different taste to it, a mildly unpleasant taste & smell.

Eventually, visitors' complaints about their water led to the decision to move. Shelley's mother, especially, had a very uncomfortable feeling that something was terribly wrong. They began the process of looking for a town with safer drinking water.

Twenty years after the family moved away from using this well, the ATSDR came short of condemning its use. The agency ordered the Town to make sure that if any family were to move onto the property again: "the new occupants should be required to connect

---

[138] "Shelley" is a fictionalized name based on the life and death of a patient I once knew but was unable to acquire permission to name her in this narrative.

immediately to the public system or to have their well sampled periodically…"[139]

Shelley, of course, showered, drank, and washed her clothes with the water that ATSDR in later years would specifically warn town officials about. During the spring and summer, the spray from the center pivots surrounding the town would moisten the community when the winds were just right. In the evenings, the fog formed by the field-sprays would hover over Bruno. Therefore, Shelley's pathways of exposure to the deadly chemicals include:

- drinking the contaminated water
- inhaling it while showering, and
- absorbing it through her skin.

Shelley was 26 years old before Nebraska established its first Natural Resource District (1982) and she would be 30 years-old (1986) before the Nebraska legislature adopted the Nebraska Chemigation Act which set penalties for chemigation infractions regarding proper center pivot equipment, such as check valves, and application usage standards.[140] By then it was already too late for Shelley. Her first symptoms were to appear two years later at age 33.

In 1973, she left home to go to college. Ten years later the Nebraska Department of Health (NDOH) initiated a 4-5-year study, conducting tests on samples from Bruno's public water supply. Those tests, completed in 1988, indicated the presence of CC14, DCA and chloroform. The NDOH was alarmed. The digging of two new wells was ordered. In the meantime, from May 1989 until October 1990, the EPA provided bottled water to the town of Bruno.[141] And so it was that Shelley had left her hometown with its **"no apparent public health hazard and indeterminate public health hazard."**

Perhaps Shelley offers us the clearest case of environmental injustice being visited upon the innocents of this world. However, her story gets worse. Shelley met Gene at the University of Nebraska in Lincoln, where he was enrolled at the School of Agriculture. Four years later (1977) they married, and Gene found a job with a Grain Storage facility in Farragut, Fremont county, Iowa, about one mile

[139] Public Health Assessment: Bruno; see "Recommendations."
[140] Nebraska Chemigation Regulations, by J. David Aiken (Lincoln: University of Nebraska, January 1992).
[141] Public Health Assessment: Bruno, (see "Background").

from Susan's family farm of her youth and two miles from Donna Jo's homestead. They found a more than adequate home directly across the street from the Grain elevator. It was almost like moving Bruno to this town!

In 1988, she and Gene had managed to scrape together enough collateral to purchase a farm about a mile outside of town (three sections to the north of Susan's home and three sections to the east of Donna Jo's). A dream had come true. There was only one problem: the water from the well tasted strangely familiar. In hindsight, a nightmare had begun!

The day they moved to the farm provided an omen of what was to come. As Shelley was putting things away into the tall shelves in the kitchen, she suddenly felt nauseated. It soon passed, leaving her feeling weak and wary. She dismissed it as simply being a factor of how her daily routine had been altered lately – including her diet, relying on fast, therefore fatty foods.

Later that evening as she and Gene lay in bed, exhausted and reviewing their day. Shelley was struck with an all-over feeling of foreboding, followed by a stabbing pain in the left side of her chest. It took her breath away as well as the other half of the thought she had been in the process of sharing with Gene. Trying to get her breath, she reached over to grip his wrist. The suddenness and the strength of her grasp startled him: "Shelley, what's wrong!"

The pain was so great she could not respond, except by intensifying her grip. Gene reached over to turn the light on. What he found was a scene he will long remember, but a scene to be repeated numerous times over the course of the next twelve years. Shelley looked as white as the bed sheets.

"My God, Shelley, what is it!"

"I…I don't know, Gene. Maybe it's just all the exertion and upset of moving. I'll be all right."

But Shelley never was all right again. She would go for weeks, months, even a year at a time with no further episodes of pain. Eventually, as the episodes increased, Gene would load her into the car for trips to the Emergency Room in Shenandoah. Subsequent tests repeatedly proved negative for anything, until the day of the 7th anniversary of their move to the farm, and the 7th anniversary of Shelley's knowing in the depths of her soul that something was wrong. It was on that day in 1995, at the age of 39, that she was finally diagnosed with breast and lung cancer.

Perhaps Shelley was NEVER: "all right"! Despite the ATSDR's diagnosis of her hometown's water, the possibility exists that the seeds of her cancer were planted in the sandbox, or by way of the family faucet, or in the shower. We will never know.

Because the conclusions of the ATSDR report were ambiguous, at best, we shall never know what really caused Shelley's cancer. All we know for sure is that Shelley died in 2000 officially of cancer of the breast with metastasis to the brain. We do know that she died protecting her family as much as possible from having to deal with the fatal prognosis, refusing any home health care because she did not want her family to see nurses around every day.

And, we know Shelley died at the age of 45 in her wheel chair while Christmas shopping for her family at a Walmart.

Chapter Six

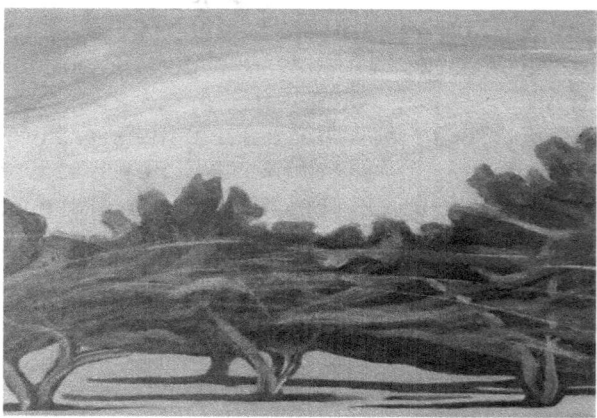

Wind Dance
By Linda Wooten-Green

Critical Analyses of Pesticide Research:
The Measure You Measure With,
Will Be Measured Back to You – and Perhaps More Besides[142]

Despite all that has been postulated here concerning the ambiguities of measurement and monitoring, there are many seemingly precise standards employed. One such standard relates to the MCLs (Maximum Contaminant Levels) considered as safe levels of exposure to a variety of chemicals. Looked at another way, any person exposed to an amount beyond the MCL would run an "unacceptable" risk of contracting the adverse health effects as listed in Appendix, Table 1.

One of the debates concerning pesticides and human health swirls around the very ability of science to make sweeping judgments about the safety levels of the chemicals. John A. Moore, who has been with the EPA's Office of Pesticides & Toxic substances claims:

The technical capability to routinely analyze in parts per million, billion, trillion, quadrillion clearly surpasses the

---

[142] An adapted version of Mark 4:24.

toxicologists' and other scientists' ability to confidently interpret human or environmental risk.[143]

Let us not forget Canadian M.D, Bruce Lanphear's claim that absolutely no pesticides are safe, NONE.[144] The inference is this:

Let's stop quibbling and simply reduce, if not stop the use altogether, of pesticides!

As C.F. Wilkinson at Cornell University's Institute for Comparative and Environmental Toxicology views the matter, "numbers add a false sense of precision and certainty," but Lanphear perhaps surprisingly, may agree with Wilkinson, at least tangentially. How so? Well, even if all the research points to some empirical level deemed to be an "acceptable level of risk," to use Wilkinson's line of argument, any declaration of safety is still based on "very imprecise, very uncertain data." In this sense, any idea of reaching any common ground for the Lanphears and the Wilkinsons would leave them each standing on shaky ground, indeed.

Furthermore, as Wilkinson points out, there is the confounding dilemma of *trans-science* – the transference or transportation of scientifically based knowledge gained from experiments on animals to the possible consequences for humans. Toxicologists are the scientists we have relied upon to inform us of the humanly safe pesticide limits – parameters established through laboratory testing of pesticides on our animal friends. Toxicology for humans can never be a precise science as long as toxicologists are limited to studies with the four-legged or the winged. Therefore:

*In the absence of rigorous experimental proof (*with human subjects*), even the best scientists are stripped of their objectivity and are reduced to making quasi-rational intuitive judgments.*[145]

The consequence for a science forced by necessity, law, ethics and morality to study the response of non-human species to

---

[143] John A. Moore, "The Not So Silent Spring," in <u>Silent Spring Revisited</u>, Gino G. Marco, ed. (Washington: American Chemical Society, 1987, 19).
[144] CF #124.
[145] Ibid, 39.

pesticides and infer parallel consequence for human life is perhaps best illustrated by a March 1998 report of the National Center for Policy Analysis (NCPA).[146] For example:

- Rodent cancer tests provide little information about how a chemical causes cancer or about low-dose risk.[147]
- "There are high-dose effects in rodent cancer tests that are not relevant to low-dose human exposures and that contribute to the high proportion of chemicals that test positive."[148]

On the other hand, while the NCPA report points out several scientific ambiguities in cancer/pesticide research, it also contributes magnificently to the climate of denial. Point Number Two of the "Executive Summary" boldly announces:

There is no epidemic of cancer, except for lung cancer due to smoking. Cancer mortality rates have declined 16 percent since 1950 (excluding lung cancer.)[149]

A special note needs to be made here: NCPA is hardly an unbiased organization. As its website states:

The NCPA's goal is to develop and promote private alternatives to government regulation and control, solving problems by relying on the strength of the competitive entrepreneurial private sector.[150]

This is an entity that will, by its nature, resist efforts by a federal or state environmental, regulatory agency to regulate the chemical industry and its products.

C.F. Wilkinson weighs in with data to support the NCPA report and to counter the idea of a cancer epidemic, by noting:

---

[146] Misconceptions About Environmental Pollution, Pesticides and the Causes of Cancer, NCPA Report No. 214 www.ncpa.org/studies/s214.

[147] Ibid, See "Misconception #7.

[148] Ibid, See "Executive Summary #3."

[149] Ibid, #2.

[150] Ibid. See "About Us."

When the trends are adjusted for the increased size of the population and for changes in age distribution the total cancer mortality rate turns out to be miniscule, especially when adjusted further for lung cancer.[151]

The issue raised in the book here is not necessarily that people are increasingly dying of cancer, but that they increasingly must live fighting it. There is no doubt that medical science has made great advances in the last 50 years learning how to destroy cancer cells or at least stall the progress of cancer.[152] At the same time, some corporations have found ways to come at it from both directions, producing products that both cause and fight cancer. See the story of Dr. Nicole Bruinsma at Chapter 10 and her dilemma while fighting a chemical company whose pesticide product may well have caused her cancer, to even consider using another product of theirs to fight her cancer.[153]

The fact is, however, people without cancer continue to acquire cancer at alarming rates. The NCPA and Wilkinson view that "there is no epidemic of cancer," because of a decline in cancer mortality, simply throws a smoke screen over the issue. The issue is two-fold: morbidity and mortality.

NCPA's position is more than a small smudge-pot on the corner of Science & Reality; it takes the form of a smokestack. Among the asserted "misconceptions" about cancer and pesticides that the NCPA Report seeks to refute are that:

- *Cancer rates are soaring.*
- *Environmental synthetic chemicals are an important cause of human cancer.*
- *Reducing pesticide residues is an effective way to prevent diet-related cancer.*
- *Identification of carcinogenic chemicals should be the primary strategy for preventing human cancer.*
- *Human exposures to carcinogens and other potential hazards are nearly all due to synthetic chemicals.*

---

[151] C.F. Wilkinson, "Being More Realistic About Chemical Carcinogenesis," www.pmep.cce.cornell.edu/facts-slides-self/facts/gen-pubre-carcin-wilkinson.
[152] See especially Mukherjee.
[153] Chapter 10, 147-149.

- *Cancer risks to humans can be assessed by standard high-dose animal cancer tests.*
- *Synthetic chemicals pose greater carcinogenic hazards than natural chemicals.*
- *The toxicology of synthetic chemicals is different than that of natural chemicals.*
- *Pesticides and other synthetic chemicals are disrupting hormones.*
- *Regulation of low, hypothetical risks is effective in advancing public health.[154]*

While the NCPA Report calls into question nearly every toxicological linkage between pesticides and human cancer, it does not directly call for epidemiological studies that would overtly and directly subject humans to the role of laboratory rats; the inference lies between the lines of each asserted "misconception." While other dynamics are at work in this report and similar ones, such as the Canadian "Report of a Panel on the Relationship Between Public Exposure to Pesticides and Cancer"[155] (See Chapter Seven), NCPA's point is well taken in noting the extent of ambiguity in a field that the general population tends to assume is very precise in its knowledge. However, NCPA succeeds only in adding to the ambiguity, even apparently attempting to misdirect future lines of scientific inquiry.

Cornell University's Breast Cancer and Environmental Risk Factors in NY State (BCERF) provides ready access to exhaustive analyses of all studies concerning the relationship between pesticides and cancer as well as other potential causes of cancer and cancer-related illness. BCERF concluded "the majority of the North American and Western European studies published since 1994 have not been able to show that white women with elevated blood or fat levels of DDE (a breakdown product of DDT) had a significantly

[154] Wilkinson, CF 151.
[155] Canadian Network of Toxicology Centres, Guelph, Ontario, Canada, Report of a Panel, Cancer 80 1997, 1887-1888. www.pmac.net/canadian ; to be cited herein as Canadian Network.

higher risk of breast cancer."[156] This statement alone may suggest many other conclusions, among them being:
1. DDE is not a problem.
2. DDT is not a problem.
3. Pesticides are not a problem.
4. WHY? Because Cornell University says so!

Look at all the Trees, But Where's the Forest?
BCERF's Critical Evaluation of Atrazine's Breast Cancer Risk[157]

After an extensive and detailed review of all research studies related to atrazine as a possible causal agent for breast cancer, BCERF concludes:

Because of the lack of case-control studies evaluating the effects of atrazine exposure on breast cancer incidence and mortality in human populations, there is insufficient evidence to conclude that atrazine is a human carcinogen.[158]

This conclusion, one might presume, is based on the strictest standards of modern science. While BCERF does call for further "human epidemiological case-control studies…to assess the risk of breast cancer…"[159] it is the conclusion cited above that gives the greatest comfort to the chemical industry.

It is indeed comforting to those who produce, distribute, and freely use the chemicals to hear a respected authority such as Cornell University note that early pesticide/cancer studies such as Dr. Donna's included no controls whatsoever. Furthermore, the chemical companies may relish noting BCERF's waving flag proclaiming that Dr. Donna (See Chapter One) "did not specifically mention that

---

[156] BCERF, "Pesticides and Breast Cancer Risk, An Evaluation of DDT and DDE, Fact Sheet #2," April 2001
www.cfe.cornell.edu/bcerf/FactSheet/Pesticide/fs2.ddt.cfm.
[157] BCERF, "Critical Evaluation #8, April 1999 www.cfe.cornell.edu/bcerf.
[158] Ibid, 127
[159] Ibid.

triazines were among the herbicides the women were exposed to (Donna, et al., 1984)"[160]

As time marched on from the Donna study, more and more studies were conducted all over the world; with more and more controls included in the matrix and design of each study. BCERF points out, for example, that a Kansas study regarding the possible link between Non-Hodgkin's Lymphoma and the triazine pesticides in 1986 by Hoar and associates included 43 controls; a Nebraska study by Zahm and associates in 1988 and Weisenberger in 1990 incorporated 725 controls.[161]

A 1997 Kentucky ecological study by Kettles and associates is faulted by BCERF for its nearly "Useless" conclusion linking breast cancer with the triazines. According to BCERF, Kettles erred by failing to define his controls more carefully. Instead of precise measurement levels of each-and-every triazine, Kettles settled for broad categories of "low, medium, and high". Furthermore, BCERF notes, Kettles offers only the ill-defined relationships of "positive and negative" between pesticide exposure and breast cancer.

Finally, BCERF points out that the Kettles study used a "surrogate measure of pesticide exposure, acres of corn planted for the years 1970, 1980 1990...such data would be expected to also predict the use of other corn herbicides..."[162]

Now, if all the studies noted above had been commissioned by BCERF, a relevant question to be raised might be: WHY BOTHER? It would seem that it is a crap shoot as to whether BCERF is going to be satisfied with any study (unless it were a study claiming safety in the use of synthetic chemicals).

The point of all studies must NOT come down to a question of whether atrazine, for example, has been proven to be a definite breast cancer carcinogen. When is enough proof enough? When is enough risk enough. There is always one more study to be done, one more gap to fill in, one more proof to one more theorem, one more control to be plugged into one more study. In the meantime, people are contracting deadly diseases, suffering and dying.

When more and more controls are built into a study, there is almost automatically a draining of the power of the data to inform us

---

[160] Ibid, 4.
[161] Ibid, 5.
[162] Ibid, 9.

of basic facts. When, for example, there are 725 controls in a given study, there is a statistical need to prove or disprove relationships between all of the variables. Soon, the study drives itself. The scientists are driven by the study, and we miss the point. The point is not whether all of the variable test out or in. The point is people are being exposed to synthesized substances in the environment, and people are getting sick, dying, and dying far ahead of their time.

BCERF's evaluation of the Kentucky study is a perfect example of the follies of factual science. Because Kettles aggregated the possibility of other pesticides into the study design, BCERF tells us that we cannot accept Kettles' conclusions pertaining to atrazine or the triazines as a group. The point that seems to become lost in the shuffle of data, the fact that gets scrambled and remains unrecognized, is the reality that all pesticides are NOT, as Dr. Bruce Lanphear concludes, good for human health. Indeed, they simply are not safe for humans. The question is not about atrazine, simazine, or Roundup. The question relates to the synthesized and cavalier use and overuse of pesticides in the food chain.

The fallacy of the studies is the underlying assumption that if you cannot prove atrazine, for example, causes NHL, then it is safe to use on our cropland, lawns, and whatever other uses the industry can dream up, leading us to believe we cannot live without it. All the while the indicting facts lie obliterated by the hype of high-powered advertising.

BCERF's critical evaluations are *critical* in every sense of the word: They appear to be "characterized by careful and exact evaluation and judgment." They are "of the nature of a crisis" – The crisis of public well-being. They are "fraught with danger or risk."[163]

It is the last sense that we need to consider at this point. BCERF's evaluations hold maximum importance due to Cornell's highly respected professional and academic reputation. Cornell's word is most often accepted as truth itself. Therefore, for a Cornell publication to state that "there is insufficient evidence to conclude that atrazine is a human carcinogen" is, in some circles, the same thing as saying "atrazine is safe," or that "atrazine is not a carcinogen" – especially in the hands of a lobbyist for the Chemical Manufacturers Association (See Chapter Seven). Cornell's

---

[163] See American Heritage Dictionary of the English Language (NY: Houghton Mifflin, 1979).

conclusion is a particularly interesting one, when we take note of the Collaborative on Health and Environment's[164] diametrically opposed statement that "atrazine may cause or at least promote ovarian cancer."[165]

According to the National Cancer Institute's report, we find the following statistics more than mildly interesting regarding Fremont County, Iowa, which was the home of the women cited in this book, a county where atrazine has been widely used:

Table 2
Female Cancer Incidence Rate* Report for Iowa[166] (Selected Cancers: State & National Averages Compared to Fremont County, Iowa)

Cancer Type	Fremont County	State of Iowa	National
Breast Cancer	177.51[167]	129.9	123.9[168]
Cancer, All Types	446.6	422.3	414.1[169]

*Rates per 100,000 population adjusted to year 2000 population.

This table suggests that women residing in Fremont County, Iowa, run a 27% higher risk of developing breast cancer than is true for the average female in the state of Iowa, and a 31% higher risk

[164] The Collaborative on Health and Environment is "a diverse network of 5,000+ individual and organizational Partners in 87 countries and 50 states, working collectively to advance knowledge and effective action to address growing concerns about the links between human health and environmental factors." www.healthandenvironment.org. Accessed August 6, 2018.
[165] Collaborative on Health and Environment, "Ovarian Cancer: What We Know," 2004. www.protectingourhealth.org/newscience/ovariancancer/ovarianknow.
[166] National Cancer Institute, "State Cancer Profiles." www.statecancerprofiles.cancer.gove/incidencerates.
[167] Rate Period: 2000-2004 (Same for Iowa).
[168] Rate Period: 2001-2004.
[169] Ibid.

than is true for the average female in the United States. Table 3 below is even more telling:

Table 3
Female Cancer Incidence & Mortality (1993-2002)[170] **(Selected Cancers and County Ranking within Iowa)[171]**

Category	Fremont County
Breast Cancer Incidence	#1
Cancer Incidence, All Types	#10
Breast Cancer Mortality	#1
Cancer Mortality, All Types	#1

* Rates per 100,000 population adjusted to year 2000 population.

The data from the above two tables also suggest that this writer's hunch, after encountering Donna Jo and the other women hospice patients in Fremont County was not far off the mark. Perhaps a cancer cluster or pocket did in fact exist. However, it is important to note Sandra Steingraber's discussion and word of caution concerning the problems associated with defining a cancer cluster, especially in an area with a population <100,000.[172] Fremont County, with a population of 7,996 in the year 2000, has been losing population ever since, down to 6,906 in 2015.

Lymphoma Foundation of America's Critical Evaluations; Studies of Pesticides and Lymphoma[173]

In contrast to BCERF'S evaluations are those of the Lymphoma Foundation of America (LFA), obviously a group dedicated to, among other things, determining the causes of lymphoma cancer

---

[170] University of Iowa, 2005 Iowa Fact Book www.public-health.uiowa.edu/Factbook/2005/CANCER.PDF.
[171] All rankings based on 99 of Iowa's 101 counties.
[172] Steingraber #1, 57-86; #2, 60-87.
[173] "Do Pesticides Cause Lymphoma?" (Chevy Chase, MD: Lymphoma Foundation of America, 2001) www.lymphomaresearch.org.

with an eye to learning how to prevent the occurrence of this and related cancers. To those ends, LFA analyzed 78 research studies related to lymphoma and pesticides. While LFA's report briefly describes each study's research design and findings as relevant to Non-Hodgkin's Lymphoma (NHL), LFA certainly makes no claim that all the studies prove a link between NHL and pesticide exposure. That is clearly not the case, and LFA notes the studies which clearly question any linkage whatsoever.

Given LFA's succinct critical evaluations, this author has taken the liberty to extrapolate some of LFA's findings. LFA does not conclude from each study that there is in fact a direct causal relationship OR a non-causal relationship between NHL and the pesticides monitored. However, a read of LFA's report leads this author to conclude that 61 of the 78 cited studies found highly suggestive causal relationships, within the limitations of their research designs:

- 08% claimed no cause-effect pattern,
- 14% were clearly neutral on the issue, leaving
- 78% with highly suggestive causal relationships.

Yet, the BCERF study of studies indicates the research has found either no relationship, or, at best, a weak relationship.[174] What?

The old adage: "If it looks like a skunk, smells like a skunk, sounds like a skunk, and feels like a skunk, then it must be a skunk," would seem to apply here. If 78% of 78 studies point to pesticides as a causal factor in incidences of a variety of cancers, then there must be something going on. If 78% of the folks I meet warn me of a potential danger lying ahead of me, I am going to assume something is going on that I need to stay away from.

A major weakness of the studies is that they generally exclude women. Nearly 60% of the studies the LFA examined dealt only with male subjects, while 3% were women only; 19% clearly included both sexes, while the remaining 18% clearly included men and MAY have included women. The most critical weakness of such studies (as well as national, state, and local regulatory policies) is the presumption of risk-benefit-cost analyses and assessments. Janette Sherman, MD, notes, "the risk-benefit language" changed in the early 1980's when "technocrats…(successfully) argued that costs

---

[174] BCERF Critical Evaluation #8, April 1999,5.

of cleanup, costs for change in technology, and costs of prevention exceeded risks;" and so it was that "risks then became 'acceptable'."[175]

The question ignored is this: For whom are the risks acceptable? Have the at-risk folks accepted the "acceptable risks" of dying at an early age? Have the young women at-risk of contracting breast cancer or ovarian cancer said it is okay if their lives are shortened, leaving behind young children? Have farmers susceptible to Parkinson's or NHL signed-off on an early sign-out with full knowledge of the pesticidal consequences for their lives? "The answer my friend," as Bob Dylan sang, "is blowin' in the wind." The answer lies, as well, in the statistics and within the human experience:

- Data released in 2016 reveal that the number of mastectomies increased by 36% from 2005 to 2013; and most were of the preventive kind. In other words, women who considered themselves to be at-risk of breast cancer, increased from 66/100,000 to 90/100,000 in choosing either a single or double mastectomy hoping to prevent an early death due to cancer.[176] Obviously, no amount of risk was acceptable for these women. They opted for precaution. Unfortunately, the precautionary option of first instance was denied to them.

- In 1982 when my youngest son, then 16, was facing the possibility of scoliosis surgery. I recall asking the surgeon, "What would be your best guess as to the consequence if the surgery is not done?" His response was immediate and chilling: "Not doing the surgery will shave-off 40 years of Brian's life." My, now 52-year-old son, could well be dead today, if we had not taken the precautionary route. The risk was just not worth it!

In other areas of public safety and public health, our regulatory agencies insist on zero tolerance for risks. There is no "acceptable risk" as far as OSHA is concerned for such things as the absence of fire extinguishers in a workplace, or the absence of

---

[175] Sherman, 25.

[176] Agency for Healthcare Research and Quality, "New Data Show Mastectomies Increased 36 Percent from 2005 to 2013," Feb 22, 2016. Accessed August 8, 2018. www.ahrq.gov/newsroom/press-releases/2016/mastectomy-sh.html

alternative exits from a building. OSHA does not care that the probability of a fire occurring might be only one in a billion. Yet, a Reasonable Maximum Exposure for Shenandoah, Iowa, according to the ATSDR, is that 557 people can be exposed to possible life-threatening chemicals, and THAT somehow, is an acceptable risk.

On the other hand, while OSHA "protects millions of people from dangerous workplace conditions," the agency made an exception for farm workers until 1992 with the passage of the Agricultural worker Protection Standard.[177] Meanwhile, the Federal Insecticide fungicide Rodenticide Act (FIFRA) mandates maximum allowable exposure levels for pesticides based on a risk-benefit analysis. The EPA, according to Earthjustice (an environmental advocacy and research organization), "uses this analysis to set exposure levels that value the appearance of produce more than the health of humans."[178] As Meriel Watts notes in her exhaustive study of the incidence of breast cancer and its relationship to pesticide exposure:

The focus should be on hazard identification and elimination, rather than risk management.[179]

SEER: Seeing What We Want to See
(The National Cancer Registry: A National Shell Game?)

Since 1973 the National Cancer Institute has been overseeing the collection of data pertaining to the incidence of cancer in the United States. This program, known as SEER (Surveillance, Epidemiology, and End results) was empowered by the National Cancer Act of 1971. SEER sounds more comprehensive than it makes any claim to be, however. The program makes no attempt to stock its database with every cancer case in the country. SEER depends on a sampling method that constitutes 14% of the populace. Currently SEER data

---

[177] "The Use of Pesticides in New Mexico," www.farmworkers.org/pestieng. Accessed March 6, 2017.

[178] Earthjustice, "Protecting Farm Workers from Pesticides," 2004 www.earthjustice.org/campaign/print.htm/?ID=09.

[179] Meriel Watts, Pesticides & Breast Cancer: A Wake Up Call (Penang, Malaysia: Pesticide Action Network [PAN Asia & the Pacific], 2007), 142.

comes from five states, plus five metropolitan areas: Connecticut, Hawaii, Iowa, New Mexico, Utah, Atlanta, Detroit, San Francisco-Oakland, Seattle, and Los Angeles. Sandra Steingraber notes:

Everyone living in one of these states or cities who is diagnosed with cancer becomes a bit of data in the SEER program registry, and their tumors stand in for all of ours.[180]

While SEER relies upon a small sampling of all incidences of cancer in the nation, it is a powerful resource with perhaps unlimited potential. SEER is not just the tabulation of cancer's prevalence but may provide an avenue to showing us the way to eradicate cancer once and for all. In Iowa in 1997 the SEER Program made it possible to provide follow-up tracking of "more than 97 percent of the 280,000 Iowans diagnosed with cancer since 1973."[181] Part of the follow-up includes several studies of specific types of cancer in Iowa, such as Non-Hodgkin's Lymphoma.

The Iowa Non-Hodgkin's Lymphoma Study (NHLS) initiated in 1997 is entitled the *Agricultural Health Study.* Together with the state of North Carolina, 89,568 adults participated[182] in the first five years of this SEER study designed to "identify occupational, environmental, dietary, and other factors that account for the excess of certain cancers among agricultural workers."[183] The NHLS includes in-home and phone interviews, the collecting of blood and cheek cell samples, pesticide and drinking water samples,[184] as well as dust samples.[185]

In addition, the Iowa State HEALTH Registry participates in the following SEER studies:

- Iowa and Missouri Radon/Lung Cancer Study[186]
- Iowa Breast Health Study

[180] Steingraber, #1, 37.

[181] Cancer Registry of Iowa – 1997 Cancer Report www.public-health.uiowa.edu/shri/annual97.

[182] Cancer Registry of Iowa – 2003 Cancer Report www.public-health.uiowa.edu/shri/annual2003.

[183] Ibid.

[184] Cancer Registry of Iowa – 1998 Cancer Report www.public-health.uiowa.edu/shri/annual98.

[185] Cancer Registry of Iowa –2000 Cancer Report www.public-health.uiowa.edu/shri/annual/00.

[186] Cancer Registry of Iowa, 2002 www.public-health.uiowa.edu/shri/annual02.

- Second Cancers Following Breast Cancer or Hodgkin's Disease
- Patterns of Care Study
- Effect of Cervical Cancer on Pregnancy Outcome
- Screening and Treatment Patterns for Breast Cancer for Healthcare Research and Quality, "New Data Show Agency Mastectomies Increased 36 Percent from 2005 to 2013," Feb 22, 2016. www.ahrq.gov/newsroom/press-releases/2016/mastectomy-sh.htmlCases
- Molecular Epidemiology Studies[187]
- Study of Cancer Survivors[188]
- Geographic Variation in Breast Cancer Treatment and Mammography Use.[189]
- Breast Cancer, Radiation Exposure, and the ATM Gene[190]
- Epidemiology of Cancer in a Cohort of Older Women – Candidate Genes for Breast Cancer[191]
- Lung Cancer Care Outcomes/Surveillance Consortium[192]

The studies noted above are only a portion of over two dozen such projects the Iowa Cancer Registry is engaged in at various stages of completion and modification. In addition, several "Data Linkage" projects such as the following are underway:

- The Quality of Cancer Surveillance Data for American Indians
- Evaluating the Cancer Incidence Experience Among a Cohort of alachlor Manufacturing Workers

---

[187] Cancer Registry of Iowa, 1997.
[188] Cancer Registry of Iowa, 1998.
[189] Cancer Registry of Iowa, 1999.
[190] No, the ATM Gene is not the gene that predetermines one's possible addiction to using ATMs. It is the gene that helps to repair damages to the DNA. However, "inheriting one abnormal ATM gene has been linked to an increased rate of breast cancer, because the abnormal gene stops the cells from repairing damaged DNA." (From: "Genetics," Breast Cancer.org, September 17, 2012 www.breastcancer.org/risk/factors/genetics.
[191] Cancer Registry of Iowa, 2000.
[192] Cancer Registry of Iowa, 2002.

- Assessments of the "Childhood Mortality and Cancer Incidence Experience of over 17,000 Children Reported by Members of the Agricultural Health Study.[193]

These studies and others are of highest importance, if we are to combat cancer. Each of these studies have been carefully executed. But despite the greatest care, methodological difficulties contribute to an on-going ambiguity in measurement and monitoring.

Much of the ambiguity inheres within SEER's routine management of its data, as noted below:

A. PLACE OF BIRTH in the SEER manual[194] allows for State only. Narrowing each state at least into regions such as rural, rural town, suburb, city and county would reward the data bank with more power.

B. ADDRESS AT FIRST SYMPTOMS & AGE AT FIRST SYMPTOMS are two categories that are NOT part of the SEER code manual but would be essential items to add at earliest possible date. Such information could lead in the long run to identifying problem areas geographically where on-set of cancer may prove to be a common experience.

C. TYPE OF REPORTING SOURCE currently allows for medical professionals, ONLY. It needs to be redefined to allow for patient/family as a type of reporting source. A common complaint among consumers of health care is that doctors do not listen to them. In this case, by honoring what patients/families report as a viable source, the medical research component would have a chance to listen.

D. TRULY FOCUS ON CANCER AS CONTRIBUTOR TO DEATH: Since SEER relies upon death certificates to certify that each death was due to cancer, SEER misses countless numbers of cancer-related deaths. Why? Simply because the "cause of death (is) often recorded as, for example, pneumonia or liver failure, when in fact the underlying cause is advanced disseminated cancer."[195]

---

[193] Cancer Registry of Iowa, 2001.

[194] SEER Manual www.public-health.uiowa.edu/shri/MAN33-55.

[195] Ralph Moss, Ph.D. "Our futile War on Cancer," New Scientist December 16, 2006 www.newscientist.com/channel/health/mg19225825.400-our-futile-war-on-cancer.

To add B and C to the SEER Manual, a whole re-evaluation of what is data and what is not needs to occur. Currently, SEER relies exclusively upon verifiable empirically-grounded medical, social and geographical data. Reportage of FIRST SYMPTOMS is largely subjective; and looked at with askance by empirical science. In many cases this information, while self-reported, would be available in the patient's medical record – particularly, AGE OF FIRST SYMPTOMS) the source relied upon by SEER examiners for information regarding "Occupation" and other items as well. Such data could provide helpful insights to at least two major issues: geography as potential source of cancer, and disease progression.

Physicians rarely inquire about the environmental conditions a patent grew up in, has/had moved in and out of, to say nothing of asking about current environmental factors.[196] These questions are understandably unasked by physicians, primarily because they see themselves as problem-solvers for individual cases of illness. How a person caught a cold, a virus, or even cancer is not the issue. The issue is the disease itself. The question is what can be done to rid this person's body of the disease. Physicians do not, in general, see themselves as medical researchers involved in preventive medicine.

On the other hand, physicians <u>are</u> medical researchers whether they want to be or not, or whether they realize it or not. Much of medical research relies upon data obtained directly and verbally from patients, as well as data obtained through trained medical observation and testing. Note, for example, the case of the SEER Program's acquisition of data – a process of gleaning data from individual medical charts.

An important observation by the President's Cancer Panel is that:

> *Physicians and other medical professionals ask infrequently about patient workplace and human environment when taking medical histories. Such information can be invaluable in discovering underlying causes of disease. Moreover, gathering this information would contribute substantially to the body of knowledge on environmental cancer risk.[197]*

---

[196] Steingraber #1, 137.
[197] <u>PCP 2010,</u> 100.

When the World Health Organization (WHO) estimates that "at least 80% of all cancer is attributable to environmental influences;[198] and when approximately 1.2 million people are newly diagnosed each year with some form of cancer, then approximately 800,000 Americans per year are walking around (if they are lucky to be able to walk) with an environmentally induced cancer. Consequently, we have over 23,000 people per 5-day work-week walking out of a doctor's office now being faced with the devastating news that they have cancer – 18,400 of whom have a cancer that may have been caused by some environmental factor.

In October 2001 three people died due to the apparent planting of anthrax in the mail. With the death of two mailroom employees, Congress became outraged at the Postal Service. The FBI, and the Center for Disease Control for being behind the proverbial eight ball in protecting the health of postal workers and the American public.[199]

Suppose we had 18,400 Americans being exposed to anthrax each week. The chances are the Federal Government would declare a National Emergency. The reality is that it is 18,400 weekly cancer victims, not 18,400 weekly anthrax victims. Somehow there is a difference. But there is no difference. These are human lives under siege, under attack, by a deadly avoidable disease.

Not long ago, a 10 page "How To" piece appeared in VOX: Science & Health offering comfort to those who have cancer, under the title of "The way we think about cancer is outdated. Here's how to change that."[200] The message conveyed is similar to the advice embedded in Bobby McFerrin's 1988 Pollyannaish hit entitled "Don't Worry, Be Happy." In other words, LIVE WITH IT!

To be fair, the author of the VOX piece is simply saying an attitude adjustment is in order. Being diagnosed with cancer is no longer an automatic death sentence. Julia Belluz points out that "the cancer death rate has dropped by 23% since 1991." She then

---

[198] Ibid. 60.
[199] Larry Lipman and Jeff Nesmith, "Anthrax strategy Assailed on Hill," Atlanta Journal Constitution, October 24, 2001, A1.
[200] Julia Belluz, "The way we think about cancer is outdated. Here's how to change that, VOX: Science & Health, March 2, 2016. www.vox.com/2016/3/2/11141452/living-with-cancer-chronic. Accessed March 6, 2016.

acknowledges that "Most of the treatments do not 'cure' the disease—instead they 'control' it, turning it into something akin to a chronic condition, like diabetes."

While I have no argument with the suggestion that cancer victims adopt a more positive outlook, I do have a problem with lulling people into thinking that cancer is just a fact of life with no regard to, or question about, cause. Furthermore, I have huge problem with a statement by one of the doctors Belluz interviewed who lumps together "thyroid, breast, prostate, and lung cancers" as simply "'pseudo-cancer...part of the aging process...not a real disease.'" The author, inadvertently, I believe, makes matters worse when she summarizes the good doctor's view as follows:

Using a different language helps patients view these concerns for what they are: an almost inevitable mutation of cells that comes with getting older.

So, as my now-deceased father-in-law, David L. Wooten, often advised, "Whatever you do, don't get old."

The medical community (medical scientists and practitioners) needs to begin raising questions ABC & D recording the answers in patients' medical records regarding their symptomatic experiences, as well as patients' thoughts regarding the why and how of contracting cancer. In this way, it would seem, medical science will have more to go on in coming to an understanding of disease progression patterns,[201] especially when there may well be differences between environmentally and non-environmentally caused cancer.

As an example, if Donna Jo, Sandra, JoAn, Susan, and Shelly's medical providers had asked the kinds of questions noted above and throughout this book, perhaps potential causal insights would have emerged in-light of the facts in Table 4 below:

All of this is to say that unless we enhance our methods of collecting cancer-related data, the ugly beast of denial will continue to thrive.

---

[201] See Sherwin Nuland, How We Die: Reflection on Life's Final Chapter(Alfred Knopf, 1994; Vintage, 1995), especially chapters entitled "The Malevolence of Cancer," and "Hope and the Cancer Patient."

Table 4. Comparative Data: Women Featured in *A Bitter Harvest*

	Age at 1ˢᵗ Symptoms	Age at DX	Age at Death
Donna Jo	40	55	58
Sandra	40	43	45
JoAn	34	38	42
Susan	28	40	41
Shelley	33	40	45

Average gap years from HS grad to 1ˢᵗ Symptoms: 17
   Range 10-22
      Average gap years from 1ˢᵗ symptoms to DX: 8
         Range: 3-15
Average gap years from DX to Death: 3
   Range: 1-5
HS Grad to DX: 25
HS Grad to Death: 28
   Range 23-40
Average gap years from 1ˢᵗ Symptoms to Death: 11.2
      Range: 5-18
NOTE: Primary Commonality: All five lived most of their lives within a range of < 1 mile (as the crow flies) to no > 5 miles from each other.

Chapter Seven

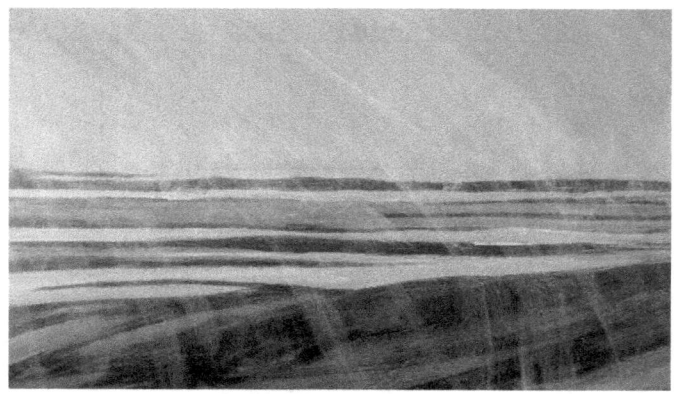

Troublesome Creek

Denial of Cancer's Environmental Causes

Regrettably, many efforts to seek concrete solutions to the environmental crisis have proved ineffective, not only because of powerful opposition but also because of a more general lack of interest. Obstructionist attitudes, even on the part of believers, can range from denial of the problem to indifference, nonchalant resignation or blind confidence on technical solutions.
(Pope Francis)[202]

To deny is "to refuse to believe." Denial is the "refusal to grant the truth of a statement or allegation."[203] Denial, like cancer, is a grievous threat to the health of a people. When the two are combined, cancer and its causal agents are the winners, being free to sow death upon humanity.

Individual & Family Denial Regarding Cancer's Environmental Causes

---

[202] Pope Francis, 14.
[203] <u>The American Heritage Dictionary of the English Language: New College Edition</u> (Boston: Houghton Mifflin, 1980).

As Elizabeth Kubler-Ross[204] explains the stages of grieving, denial is a normal response to loss. In fact, after the initial shock of being informed by one's physician that a person has cancer, patients commonly deny the diagnosis:

- "No, there must be some mistake. They must have my x-rays mixed up with someone else's!"
- "I'll beat it!"
- "That doctor never knew what he/she was doing, anyway. What the (bleep) does he/she know about it?"

Kubler-Ross has observed that denial is a "healthy way of dealing with the uncomfortable and painful…usually a temporary defense…"[205] At some point most people diagnosed with a terminal disease are able to move to some level of acceptance. The journey from denial to acceptance can be long or short, emotionally excruciating or a brief "blip" on the radar screen of life. The process almost always engages many questions with fee answers. One of those questions is: "How did this happen?" Another is: "Why?"

Over two decades and a half ago, my first wife, Dawn, died of ovarian cancer at the age of 51. Other than some fleeting thoughts connecting her cancer to her childhood bout with leukemia, neither of us spent much time asking the "how" question. There was little time. There was little energy. There was the cancer and we had to deal with its ugliness in our life. We did not have the resources or the imagination to entertain the possibility of an environmental cause. Besides, any such issue would be moot. Dawn was dying.

Soon after her death, a close friend and former work associate from our years in Casper, Wyoming, called to inform me that she, too, had been diagnosed with ovarian cancer at age 45. In the middle of a sometimes-tearful conversation, Margo asked "what is in the water in Casper, Ron?"

Margo had journeyed from denial to acceptance to hope – the hope that someday, someone would find the cause, opening-up the possibility of prevention. It was already too late for Margo; she was dying, but her plea was that others be spared. "There is something out there," she said, "And something has to be done." This book is, in part, a response to Margo's plea.

---

[204] Elizabeth Kubler-Ross, On Death and Dying (NY: Macmillan, 1969).
[205] Ibid, 35-36.

Community Denial: Cancer & Environmental Causes

An entire community may exhibit denial. At the national level, we as a nation seem to hold the attitude that cancer is just a fact of life. It is simply a part of the human condition. This attitude does not deny that cancer is a problem of some magnitude. Rather, it is an attitude shared with the often-held view about death and taxes: there is nothing we can do about it. We just need to hope and pray our number does not come up. Perhaps we need to hope for luck as "when the guy next to you gets hit with the arrow."[206]

Some avoid the arrow of cancer. Some acquire a longer lease on life after the diagnosis. Some even beat it. However, **as a society** we have largely resigned ourselves to the fatalistic view that cancer is probably going to get us, unless we are lucky. We have become like the proverbial frog in the pot of boiling water, accepting the gradually increasing temperature as normal. We seriously doubt that cancer can be avoided, an unholy marriage of denial and acceptance. We do hope for a miracle, a miracle cure, a miracle turn-around of the incidences of cancer. Until then, however, we hold to the "truth" that:

...there is nothing to be done except slice off women's breasts, pump their bodies full of toxic chemicals to kill cancer cells, burn them with radiation, and bury our dead.[207]

Despite some members of the town of Bruno taking the initiative to express their concerns leading to the ATSDR study, only 12 out of the 170 community residents attended a public meeting facilitated by ATSDR staff on March 17, 1993.[208] An eight percent turnout, by some standards may be considered expressive of concern. By any standard, it should not be labeled as denial of a community-wide problem. Such a turnout, on the other hand, may be regarded as denial that anything will get done. With only 12 people out of 170 attending, must surely have been a disappointment to those in the

---

[206] Ernest Becker, The Denial of Death (The Free Press, 1997, 2).
[207] Peter Montague, "What Causes Breast Cancer?" 2001. www.toxics.net/breastcancer.html.
[208] Public Health Assessment: Bruno; See "Community Health Concerns."

community who took the initiative that spurred ATSDR's assessment.

The fact that 92% of the people stayed home that evening may be deemed a measure of apathy. If so, the Apathy or Fatalism Factor rose to its maximum level between June 30 and July 29, 1994 when not one comment was received by ATSDR during the public comment period regarding the agency's published report.[209] Behind most apathy, however, is the sense that my voice, my vote, my presence does not matter; or the more cynical attitude that its all a farce, so why bother? The result, once again, is the communal sanctioning of the unholy marriage of denial and acceptance: things are as they always have been and will remain ever so. "It is what it is." Fundamentally, this sometimes-well-founded public attitude comes down to a disease of the body politic, a feeling of helplessness and political insignificance.

On the other hand, in most communities the incentives for maintaining a posture of denial remain. In a rural community where the farmers who sustain the town's economy depend upon the ready availability of pesticides at the local Agrico Supply, and Agrico is the biggest employer in town, second only to the school district, the act of even raising the questions about pesticides as a cause of cancer can be much more than the local economic and emotional traffic can bear.

A case in point is that of Wisconsin State Representative Gary Hebl's aborted attempt to introduce a bill which would have "banned the distribution and sale of all herbicides that contain atrazine in the State...[210] Apparently Rep. Hebl heard from too many farmers to risk going through with his proposed legislation.

Economic dependency breeds and feeds denial. The cruel fact is that rural communities can become so dependent on pesticide use, pesticide availability, pesticide-based income, and pesticide-related employment that a form of socially prescribed behavior sets in. As an individual diagnosed with lung cancer due to smoking continues lighting up and inhaling his/her three packs a day, the chemically dependent rural community will naturally and understandably

---

[209] Ibid. (See "Public Health Actions.")
[210] Wisconsin Ag Connection, "Hebl Decides to Drop Legislation to Ban Atrazine in Wisconsin," (February 18, 2010).
www.wisconsinconnection.com/Story-State.php?Id=202.

continue "lighting up, inhaling and ingesting" their triazines each day.

Such economically dependent communities are, in effect, addictive organizations, displaying all of the characteristics of the addictive personality and the addictive family, not least of which is the tendency toward denial. The addictive personality will deny to the very end that he/she has an addiction to alcohol or cigarettes or gambling or whatever the addiction may be. Family members tend to support the addiction by publicly denying the problem, keeping secrets, covering up and making excuses. An addicted community[211] will also support the addiction be keeping its own secrets, covering up and making excuses/justifications. An addicted community may, on the other hand, have a clear view of the problems, but also hold to a defeatist attitude: "What choice do we have!"

In addition, there is a tyranny that pervades and controls the addicted community. This tyranny maintains itself through the power of fear:

- the fear of offending one's neighbors and friends and relatives by questioning the generally accepted, the unquestionable;
- the fear that comes from knowing very intuitively that to raise such questions is to invite reprisal from the power structure within the community; and
- the fear of being ostracized.

    In such an environment of dependency and fear, denial and/or avoidance is a natural response.

Governmental Denial: Cancer & Environmental Causes

For over 40 years the Pentagon denied that US Navy personnel (without their consent or knowledge) were intentionally exposed to "live biological warfare agents" during the 1960's and 1970's. Finally, in October 2001, the Pentagon admitted to the existence of "Project SHAD—Project Shipboard Hazard and Defense," while

---

[211] The characteristics of an addicted community would be very similar to those of the addictive organization described in The Addictive Organization: Why We Overwork, Cover Up, Pick Up the Pieces, Please the Boss and Perpetuate Sick Organizations, by Anne Wilson Schaef & Diane Faisel (Harper, 1990).

denying any harmful effects to the servicemen and women involved.[212] Project SHAD is but one example of government denial preventing the proper assessment of and care for the health and welfare of its citizens.

Similarly, the EPA and medical scientists had been aware for at least 10 years that atrazine had been banned in Austria, Germany, Hungary, Italy, Netherlands, Norway, Sweden, and other countries as well; yet, atrazine continued to be loaded onto American land, food, and people.[213] In 1984 Dr. A. Donna established the statistical correlation between such triazines as atrazine and the occurrence of ovarian cancer among women farmers in Northern Italy.[214]

The President's Cancer Panel quotes Dr. Tyrone Hayes, a professor of Integrative Biology at University of California, Berkeley, who laments:

We use 80 million pounds (of atrazine) annually in the United States. It's the number-one pesticide contaminant of ground water, surface water, and drinking water. It's used in more than 80 countries, but it's now outlawed in all of Europe or, as the company likes to say, has been denied regulatory approval. The main point here is that here's a compound that we use 80 million pounds of, and it's illegal in the home country (Switzerland) of the company (Syngenta) that makes it.[215]

Yet, the EPA and many in the American medical science establishment continue to deny that atrazine had been linked in powerfully significant ways as a drinking water pollutant or as a cause of cancer.[216] Even repeated evidence presented to the EPA by independent monitoring organizations that weed killers in tap water are alarmingly exceeding EPA's own "cancer risk benchmark," was

---

[212] Mark Pazniokas and Dennis Williams (Hartford Current), "Navy admits what crews knew: Tests biological," Atlanta Journal Constitution, October 21, 2001, A21.

[213] Fagan, 21.

[214] A. Donna, et al, "Triazine Herbicides and Ovarian Epithelial Neoplasms, Scandinavian Journal of Work Environments and Health 15 1989: 47-53; See also: "Ovarian Mesothelial Tumors and Herbicides: A Case-Control Study," Carcinogenesis 5 (1984): 941-42.

[215] PCP 2010, 46.

[216] Fagan, 21.

largely ignored or denied as a problem.[217] Could it be that the foxes are "guarding" the henhouse? (See Chapter eight).

Have we truly gone over the edge of morality and ethics, as Thomas Hartmann suggests in his realistically cynical analysis of the political, economic and moral consequences of public policy?

(T)here's no question that asbestos is good for economic growth. Indeed, every cancer avoided is a quarter-million-dollars lost to the medical service part of our economy – which is today about one-seventh of the entire economy. Similarly, economic activity is reduced by regulations that reduce cancer-causing arsenic in drinking water, or soot from power plants, and auto exhaust, or emissions of chemicals from factories, exposures to pesticides and other agricultural chemicals by farm workers and consumers.[218]

Medical Denial: Cancer & Environmental Causes

Despite millions of people who have died of cancer and the millions who are currently under treatment for cancer, there are those in the medical world who deny any notion of a cancer epidemic. For example, the NCPA and the Canadian Panel cited previously, plus C.F. Wilkinson of Cornell University (See Chapter 5) have all claimed in their own ways that "absolutely no evidence exists that we are in the midst of a human cancer epidemic."[219]

NCPA, in fact, makes the further claim that:

There is no convincing epidemiological evidence, nor is there much toxicological plausibility, that the levels of DDT normally found in the environment are likely to be a significant contributor to cancer.[220]

---

[217] Brian A. Cohen, Tough to Swallow: How pesticide companies profit from poisoning America's tap water

[218] Thomas Hartmann, What Would Jefferson Do?: A Return to Democracy (Harmony Books, 2004), 108.

[219] Silent Spring Revisited, 41; See also NCPA Report and Canadian Network.

[220] NCPA Report #7.

And:

There is no convincing evidence that synthetic chemical pollutants are important for human cancer.[221]

Indeed, the entire thrust of the report from the Canadian Network of Toxicology Centres is that of a denial of any relationship between public exposure to pesticides and cancer. All that the Canadian report admits is that lung cancer is related to tobacco smoking and that those who handle pesticides have indeed contracted cancer. On the other hand, the Canadian panel of experts does call for on-going research regarding the possible link between cancer and pesticides.

Whether it is denial, avoidance, or willful over-looking, the Canadian Panel's number one conclusion causes one to question the entire report's reliability:

Concerns have been raised that pesticide exposure may be an important cause of cancer. The Panel was unaware of any direct evidence developed since the Doll and Peto assessment in 1981 to suggest any major revision of their view that synthetic sources of chemicals are responsible for only a small percentage of all cancer mortality.[222]

Again, we are not focused exclusively herein with the issue of cancer-related mortality. Rather, we are more concerned about cancer-related morbidity and the millions of people who are diagnosed with cancer each year.

Dennis T. Avery, Senior Fellow at the Hudson Institute and director of the Center for Global food Issues, adds to the apparent chorus of denial as he intones the question: "Do pesticide residues cause cancer?" His answering refrain:

We've added 30 years to our life spans in the 20th Century, eight of them since we started spraying pesticides widely…. After

---

[221] NCPA Executive summary #4.
[222] Canadian Network, 16.

billions of dollars spent trying, not one pesticide-residue cancer victim has been found.[223]

These conclusions are reached despite the numerous studies noted herein, especially Dr. Donna's 1984 study and the many studies cited by Steingraber. In addition, the Canadian Panel concludes that while "pesticide residues have been detected in drinking water," pesticides are "not found to be an important route of exposure…" The problem with this conclusion is that it is based on the EPA's Non-Occupational Pesticide Exposure Study (NOPES) of only two cities.[224] Since NOPES is a non-occupational exposure study, it would have been well for the EPA to include the Cape Cod experience, described below, in its research design.

The Cape Cod Project:
A Geographic Information System (GIS)

Due to a growing awareness of high incidences of breast cancer among women on Cape Cod, the Silent Spring Institute (SSI), named in honor of Rachel Carson, launched a massive research effort known as the Cape Cod Breast Cancer and Environment Study deploying a Geographic Information System (GIS). The GIS is designed to "study the relationship between residential exposure to pesticides and breast cancer on Cape Cod." Recorded data regarding pesticide use from 1948 to 1995, as well as meteorological information, proximity to residential locations, and many other variables are entered into the GIS computer program capable of estimating a person's risk of exposure to carcinogens, and risk of contracting cancer.[225]

---

[223] Dennis T. Avery, "Why Greens Should Love Pesticides," The Wall Street Journal, August 12, 1999. www.highyieldconservation.org/articles/greens_love-pesticides.

[224] Cf. 53 at Ibid, 11 & 20.

[225] See Silent Spring Review, Winter 2002 (Silent Spring Institute), 5; and JG Brody, et al, "Using GIS and historical records to reconstruct residential exposure to large-scale pesticide application," www.ncbi.nlm.nih.gov/entrez/query.fcgi?cmd=Retrieve&db=PubMed&list_uids=1185943.

GIS is certainly not an infallible tool. The availability of essential data defines its limitations. After reviewing local and state government pesticide regulatory documents as well as survey research and focus group results, SSI decided to focus initially on large-scale tree pest control, cranberry cultivation, and golf course turf management."[226]

When necessary data are available, SSI's Spatial Proximity Tool (SPT), an added component to GIS, classifies specific locations as "exposed" or "unexposed" on a scale of relative intensities of exposure. Utilizing data such as historical records of wind velocity and aerial spraying, SSI's Geographic Information System and its Spatial Proximity Tool can assess the degree of pesticide/cancer exposure a person has accrued simply by residing at a specific location over time.[227]

SSI's Cape Cod Study advances the science of assessing Multiple Chemical Sensitivity (MCS). Until the Cape Cod Study came along, MCS was considered a function of one person's sensitivity to multiple exposures of one chemical at one historical moment. Only rarely has there been any consideration to one person's multiple exposures to multiple chemicals; and then the considerations have been limited to one historical exposure moment of event. The GIS SPT can calculate risk data for many people in one geographic location over an extended-period. SSI's study:

...estimated the relative intensities of pesticide exposures between 1948 and 1995 at each of the 2,100 study participants' Cape residences. During these years, more than two-dozen chemicals...were used on cranberry bogs and other agricultural land, wetlands, forests, golf courses, and rights-of-way. Cape residents living in or near these areas may have been exposed at the time of spraying and, over time, to residues in soil, food crops, or drinking water.[228]

---

[226] JG Brody, et al, "Using GIS and historical records to reconstruct residential exposure to large-scale pesticide application," Journal of Exposure analysis and Environmental Epidemiology 2002, 66.

[227] Ibid, 12, 64-80.

[228] "New Computer Tool Assesses Women's Pesticide Exposures," Silent Spring Institute, Press Release, February 27, 2002.

Unfortunately, the Massachusetts Department of Health chose not to fund soil sampling or the testing of ground and drinking water in Phase Two of the Cape Cod study.[229] The results have been somewhat tenuous due to "uncertainties"[230] associated with the exposure assessments. No significant relationship has been shown to exit between pesticide use and breast cancer. However, "after controlling for established breast cancer risk factors," the Cape Cod Study has found that "living longer on Cape cod is significantly associated with higher breast cancer risk..."[231]

Now, as of December 2017, that which was initiated by SSI's GIS program has taken on a new life with funding through 2022 provided by the STEEP Superfund Program Research Center. The STEEP funding will include testing of private water wells for PFASs (highly chlorinated chemicals). Currently, there are over 3000 such chemicals, some of which have been linked to cancer.[232] Scientists from SSI, Harvard University and the University of Rhode Island are providing expertise and leadership.

NEPHTN:
The National Environmental Public Health Tracking Network

The Cape Cod Study has proven the necessity and feasibility of a nationwide monitoring system, one that is more expansive and accurate than the National Cancer Registry. To that end, Congress funded the formation of a National Environment Health Tracking System in March 2002,[233] now known as the National Environmental

---

[229] Julia Green Brody, Joel Tickner, and Ruth Ann Rudel, "Community-Initiated Breast Cancer and Environment Studies and the Precautionary Principle," Environmental Health Perspectives (The National Institute of Environmental Health Sciences, National Institute of Health and Human Services, August 2005) www.ehp.niehs.nih.gov-member.
[230] Ibid, 21.
[231] Ibid.
[232] "Scientists Kick Off Research Center Focused on Cape cod Drinking Water Contaminants," December 6, 2017. www.capecod.com/newscenter/scientists-kick-off-research-center-focused-on-cape-cod-drinking-water-contaminats.
[233] "Bill Introduced to Improve Environmental Health Tracking," Beyond Pesticides Daily News Archive, March 25, 2002. www.beyondpesticides.org/NEWS/daily_news_archive/03_25_02.htm.

Public Health Tracking Network (NEPHTN), a service provided by the Center for Disease Control in Atlanta, Georgia.

NEPHTN builds upon existing tracking systems such as SEER, the National Health Interview Survey (NHIS), the National Hospital Discharge Survey (NHDS), and the National Ambulatory Medical Care Survey (NAMCS), while recognizing that they each provide useful information regarding certain public health issues, and yet, "were not designed…to pinpoint clusters of chronic disease and link them to communities exposed to environmental contaminants."[234]

"If only we had known!"

If, in 1945, fourteen years before Shelley was born, when the U.S. Fish and Wildlife Service issued their first alert concerning the deleterious effects of DDT;

- Or, 17 years later when Rachel Carson's book, <u>Silent Spring</u> expanded the warning (and Shelley was 7);
- Or, if in 1984 when Dr. Donna's study in Northern Italy was published, action had been taken to ban DDT and the triazines from the market,

Would it have made a difference for Shelley, or any of the other people chronicled herein?

We, of course, do not really know.

Shelley was 29 years old at the time of Dr. Donna's report. She had already lived most of her life in rural towns surrounded by cropland where atrazine was one of the pesticides of choice, pesticides that had impacted the land, the water and even the air she breathed. Four years after the Donna study came out, Shelley and Gene bought their farm. Perhaps it was already too late for any of the women mentioned here, but what about their children? Their children's children?

Sadly, we **were** warned! In 1962 Rachel Carson cautioned all who would listen:

---

[234] "Chronic Disease Tracking Fact Sheet," The Children's Environmental Health Institute (www.cehi.org/chronicdisease.htm. See also: http://ephtracking.cdc.gov. Accessed August 15, 2018.

We have put poisonous and biologically potent chemicals indiscriminately into the hands of persons wholly ignorant of their potential for harm. We have subjected enormous numbers of people to contact with these poisons, without their consent, and often without their knowledge.[235]

Perhaps now, like Project SHAD, we are coming to realize 50+ years after the initial "whistle" was blown that there **was** a problem all along. Environmental and medical researcher Sandra Steingraber observes it is extremely rare that a cancer patient is asked about "environmental conditions" where they have grown and lived.[236] Yet, nearly 75% of all cancers are estimated to be environmentally caused.[237]

It is the exploration of environmental conditions associated with the geography of birthplace and proposing some answers to the questions never asked of cancer patients that provide much of the focus of this book. In pursuit of answers to the unasked questions, it is hoped that we can break through the problem of pervasive personal, public, political, and professional denial.

All things considered, it should not be difficult to end the denial concerning whether pesticides are a causal agent for breast cancer. Especially for women. Meriel Watts of New Zealand and the Pesticide Action Network of Malaysia have published an exhaustive and persuasive study of the extant evidence that pesticides create "killing fields"[238] throughout the world.

Watts examines 101 pesticides (organochlorines, triazine herbicides, fungicides, other pesticides, inerts and contaminants). These chemicals are presented together with eight markers related to

---

[235] Carson, 12.

[236] Steingraber #1, 137.

[237] Lichtenstein, P., et al, "Environmental and heritable factors in the causation of cancer – analyses of cohorts of twins from Sweden, Denmark, and Finland," New England Journal of Medicine, 2000. 343(2): 78-85.

This study "combined data on 44,788 pairs of twins listed in the Swedish, Danish, and Finish Twin Registries... Statistical modeling was used to estimate the relative importance of heritable and environmental factors."

A cautionary note: The term *environment* in the Lichtenstein study is very broadly defined and does not necessarily include nor preclude pesticides, pollution, or the like.

[238] "Killing fields" in this case is my term, not a term used by Dr. Watts.

potential risks as cancer causing gents indicated by dozens of scientific studies. The markers note whether a given pesticide has been statistically associated with being carcinogenic in: breast cancer epidemiology, mammary tumors, estrogenic activity, other hormonal effects, immune system disruption, mammary gland development, evidence of carcinogenicity, and GJIC[239] inhibition.[240]

To make a long statistical story short, the following analysis is based on Watts' table of data where she has carefully and simply noted with a plus sign (+) for each pesticide within a grid of the corresponding matrix of eight markers whether a given pesticide has been found to be associated with breast cancer.

My extrapolation of Dr. Watts' tabular data would render a 100%, if a given pesticide has been found to be a potential for increasing the risk of breast cancer across all markers. A 0% would indicate that a given pesticide has not as yet, risen to the level of any statistically grounded risk for causing breast cancer.

In that vein, it is most instructive and alarming that all 14 organochlorines present themselves as having at least one area for potential breast cancer risk, and that includes all of the organochlorines mentioned in the current book. For example, DDT/DDE (88%). Chlordane/endosulfan/methoxychlor/toxaphene (76%), heptachlor/lindane (63%), dieldrin/HCB (50%). All others in the organochlorine class register between 25-38%; not one scores a 0%.

In the case of triazine herbicides, atrazine ranks with DDT/DDE at 88%, fenvalerate at 75%, cyanazine/propazine/simazine produce a 38% risk, and all others in this class come in at 13-25%; again, not one registers a 0%.

One wonders, what more does it take to end the denial? Realistically, however, breaking through denial is one thing; breaking through collusion and complicity is quite another task.

---

[239] GJIC=Gap Junctional Intercellular Communications. According to the American Society of Clinical Oncology, GJIC "is required for embryonic development, tissue homeostasis and cell proliferation. It has been repeatedly emphasized that gap junction proteins connexins (CXS) are defective in most human malignancies and that their alteration may play a role in carcinogenesis." From: "Intercellular Communication and Prostate Carcinogenesis," www.asco.org/portal/site/ASCOv2/template.RAW/menuitem.alc60e3.

[240] See ""Table 3: Summary of evidence of potential to increase breast cancer risk" in Watts, 135-138; or request copies at wootengreen@msn.com.

Chapter Eight

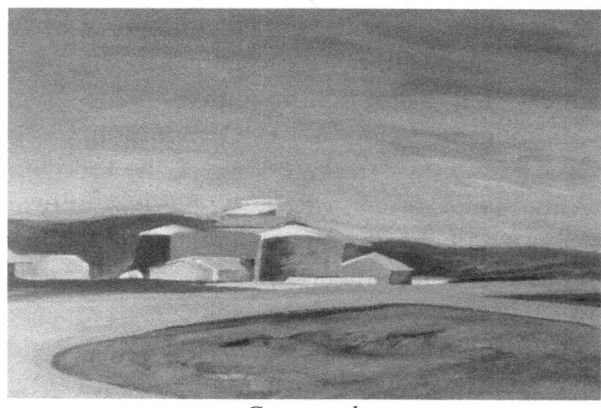

Crossroads
By Linda Wooten-Green

Co-optation: Expertise vs. Collusion

Many of those who possess more resources and economic or political power seem mostly to be concerned with masking the problems or concealing their symptoms…
(Pope Francis)[241]

The Co-optation of Government Agencies:

In early May 1999 seven of the eleven members of EPA's Tolerance Reassessment Advisory Committee (TRAC) resigned citing White House and EPA "lack of action while bowing to pesticide and agribusiness pressure and demands."[242] Delay tactics such as ever-lengthy debates were cited as among the strategies that led to the mass resignation. The seven dissenters did not directly charge that the Clinton Administration or the EPA had colluded with the pesticide/agribusiness camp, but the implication was clear.

TRAC had been formed a year earlier to help EPA with its implementation of the food Quality Protection Act. Its members represented the American Crop Protection Association, Monsanto Company, Novartis Crop Protection, Dow Agro Sciences, *Natural*

---

[241] Pope Francis, 26.
[242] Endocrine Disruptor News Archive: January-June 1999.

Resources Defense Council, Consumers Union, Pesticide Education Center, World Wildlife Fund, Farm Workers Justice Fund, National Campaign for Pesticide Policy Reform, C.A.T.A. Farm Worker Support Committee.

Those who resigned are highlighted above in *Italics.* It requires no extraordinary genius to note that those who resigned from TRAC were the activist, environment-oriented members most likely to want immediate action. Those remaining represented corporate interests with a greater economic stake in maintaining the status quo.

Jeff Stier, Associate Director of the American Council on Science and Health (ASCH) described the departed organizations as having "an anti-technology bias." Their call for a "ban of these safe pesticides," he believed, "would jeopardize the quality and increase the price of produce."[243]

It appears that one side of TRAC's table was concerned about "safe pesticides," while the other was concerned about securing safe foods. Despite the apparent chasm separating the two sides, there is a common ground. Both seek "quality" food, but that is the extent of their common vision. As the cliché goes, "the devil is in the details." The "details" in defining "quality" represent a great divide.

The corporate side is interested in securing their financial interests as any business would. They are seeking greater and greater sales and profits while believing that those goals will also satisfy the gols of increased production of quality food. More and more quality food will be found in the cupboards of American homes while increasing profits for farmers, processors, retailers and distributors alike.

The activist/environmentalist side is interested in securing that foodstuffs, land, air, and water are free of disease-inducing, life-threatening chemicals for the farmer, field worker, processor, distributor, and consumer. They inherently skeptical of the agrichemical claims of safe and secure chemicals. As Steir suggests, the corporate side is equally suspicious of those who respond to the latest advances in technology with an apparent knee-jerk negativism.

It must be noted that TRAC's last meeting was held in October 1999. Soon afterward EPA and USDA established a new advisory panel known as the Committee to Advise on Reassessment

---

[243] Ibid.

and Transition (CARAT). CARAT's charge was "to provide advice on strategic approaches for pest management planning, transition, and tolerance reassessment for pesticides as required by the Food Quality Protection Act (FQPA).[244] It appears that CARAT's last meeting may or may not have been held on July 17-18, 2003. However, no transcript is publicly available as of the last webpage update on February 26, 2011.[245]

The trials of TRAC illustrate a general and very common problem of government – the co-optation of administrative agencies by special interest groups. The regulating banks, agriculture, education, tend to be administered by bankers, agriculturalists, educators respectively. Co-optation is a fact of political life with certain advantages: namely those who know something about the activity itself administer that area of governing. However, co-optation often comes at a price: namely the price of self-aggrandizement for special interests at a cost to public welfare and the general good.[246]

When President George W. Bush named Linda J. Fisher, a former Monsanto Company executive as his choice for EPA Deputy Administrator, environmental groups such as Beyond Pesticides took immediate note with alarm.[247] Now, in the present American political climate, we witness full-scale, "full-court-press" attempts to implement and legitimate "overt cooptation" with "covert encroachment by external interests on organizational power which deflects organizational activity from its intended goal."[248] See AFTERWORD.

---

[244] U.S. Environmental Protection Agency & U.S. Department of Agriculture Tolerance Reassessment Advisory Committee of the National Advisory Council for Environmental Policy and Technology. www.epa.gov/oppfead1/trac.

[245] www.epa.gov/pesticides.carat. Accessed July 1, 2015.

[246] See Les Metcalfe's "Flexible Federalism," Comparative Perspective (Indiana University, Bloomington, Indiana (47405 5-8 April 1997), for an extensive analysis of the dynamics of Co-optation with the starting point being "The classic analysis of cooptation" by Selznick's study of "The TVA and the Grassroots" (1949).

[247] "Bush Names Former Monsanto Executive as Deputy Administrator," Beyond Pesticides Daily News Archive, March 29, 2001 www.beyondpesticides.org/NEWS/daily_news_archive/03_29_01.htm.

[248] www.indiana.eedu/cstc/metcalf1 (Accessed June 20, 2003. NOTE: As of February 15, 2016, this paper no longer appears to be available on the web.

The Co-optation of Environmental Organizations

While the focus of this book is, among other things, upon the relationship between the pesticide industry and government, it would be a major oversight if we ignored one other important dimension of co-optation, namely the co-opting of environmental organizations by the pesticide industry. Some environmental organizations have allowed themselves to be not only heavily influenced by "the enemy," but have apparently been drawn into becoming "partners in crime."

<u>The Case of the Nature Conservancy</u>

The Nature Conservancy describes itself as:

...the leading conservation organization working around the world to protect ecologically important lands and waters for nature and people[249].

Soon after the Nature Conservancy established its Texas chapter, one of its top priorities was to protect and save Attwater's Prairie Chicken. One of the few surviving breeding grounds, at the time, was located on 2000+ acres along Galveston Bay. In 1995 Mobile Oil Company, the owner of this tract of land, which had seen many oil rigs, announced it as donating the land to The Nature Conservancy. Why? Well, as Mobile said at the time, it would be:

The last best hope of saving one of the world's most endangered species.[250]

Four years later in 1999, the Conservancy retained an oil and gas company to move onto the Texas City Prairie Preserve to "sink a new gas well inside the preserve." Why? To obtain funds for pursuing the organization's mission.[251] It took about three years

---

[249] http://www.nature.orrg/about-us/index.htm?intc=nature.tnav.about. Accessed March 17, 2015.
[250] Klein, 192.
[251] Ibid.

before, shall we say, the "Texas Nature Conservancy Oil Company," became a controversy. It was then that the Conservancy appeared to spread its wings in the shape of a truly co-opted organization. The Conservancy, like all gas and oil drilling companies, defended its gas drilling operation by claiming:

We can do this drilling without harming the prairie chickens and their habitat.[252]

We now know the Nature Conservancy receives funding support from Shell and BP. However, the relationship goes beyond financial support and even membership. BP America, Chevron, and Shell are represented on the Conservancy's Business Council.[253] In addition, the former CEO of Duke Energy currently sits on the Conservancy's board of directors as Vice Chair, along with the Chairman and CEO of Dow Chemical Co & Director of DowDuPont.[254]

Other environmental organizations whose membership, leadership, and financial support Rises questions concerning just how far they can go action-wise without making their corporate "sugar daddies" nervous and down-right rebellious. For example:

- Conservation International (CI) whose largest contributor is Monsanto Corporation,[255] and
- The International Agency for Research on Cancer (IARC), which has been infiltrated by chemical companies.[256]

---

[252] Ibid, 193.

[253] Ibid, 196.

[254] http://www.nature.org/about-us/governance/board-of-directors/index.htm. Accessed August 21, 2018.

[255] Klein, 196.

[256] Jon Luoma, "Under the Influence: Is industry becoming an inside player at the world's leading research center on carcinogens?" (NRDC, OnEarth, Fall 2002. www.nrdc.org/onearth/02fal/iarc.asp.

Collusion Pollution

To collude is to act with others in such a way as to deceive yet others. While the trial of TRAC noted earlier are trials of co-optation, they ring of the possibility of collusion, i.e., that some of the actors involved were acting in concert with each other to deceive yet other members of TRAC. The departing members of TRAC allude to certain improprieties, but all of that may be nothing more than illusion.

Collusion does not have to be actions agreed to in smoke-filled rooms by nefarious characters scheming to destroy others for personal gain. Collusion can be and, perhaps, normally is much subtler. The literature indicates a subtle collusive movement toward a total discounting of pesticide toxicology's reliance on rodents and rabbits, and a fervent call for epidemiological testing of pesticides on humans. Let us examine the flow of argumentation:

J.E. Davies and R. Doon made one of the earlier attempts at bringing up the need for more directly valid studies of the human response to pesticide exposure as opposed to the more indirect conclusions drawn from toxicology's observations in animal labs. Davies, at the time (1987) was with the University of Miami's School of Medicine's Department of "Epidemiology and Public Health and Environment, Port-of-Span, Trinidad-Tobago, West Indies. While noting how early toxicology studies found links between pesticides and cancer in animals tested in laboratories, extrapolated to consequences for human health, Davies and Doon observe:

...in the last decade (1997-1987) epidemiologic studies have on the whole been reassuring because pesticide-linked carcinogenesis has not been widely proven....[257]

Subsequent epidemiological apologias have dismissed the toxicology of pesticides. The NCPA report on "Misconceptions About Environmental Pollution, Pesticides and the causes of cancer" off-handedly notes how the "assumption that synthetic chemicals are Hazardous has led to a bias in testing…" The argument is then taken

---

[257] J.E. Davies and R. Doon, "Human Health Effects of Pesticides," <u>Silent Spring Revisited</u>, 117-118.

directly to how the "natural world of chemicals has never been tested systematically."[258] While obliquely dismissing toxicology's findings, this argument diverts attention away from the human health consequences of humanly produced chemicals toward a fascination with chemicals found in the natural environment produced by Mother Nature herself. The NCPA argument comes to its fulfillment with the conclusion that:

Our results call for a reevaluation of the utility of animal cancer tests in protecting the public against hypothetical risks.[259]

The composition of NCPA's Board of Directors provides an additional clue to the slant of the organization. With Chairman of NCPA's Board, James Cleo Thompson, Jr., who is with Thompson Petroleum Corporation, and Peter DuPont as a board member, the chances are especially slim that NCPA would ever approve of governmental regulation of chemicals.

Was there collusion in the preparation of NCPA's Report #214 examining the "misconceptions" surrounding pesticide causes of cancer? Perhaps not, but the values, goals, purpose, worldview, and economic interests of NCPA, its Board members, and membership at-large would naturally define the nature of NCPA'S findings.

As a further example, let us note Gustave Kohn's investigative report entitled "Agriculture, Pesticides and the American Chemical Industry."[260] After allowing that Rachel Carson was a "prophet," Kohn goes on to Paint her "present-day disciples" as "less discerning…more strident. They may well obstruct the future of both science and our nation's economic development."

Obstruct the future of both science and our nation's economic development?

This charge, that any effort to control or possibly ban the use of pesticides would obstruct "our nation's economic development" dramatically illustrates one of Naomi Klein's central theses in This

---

[258] NCPA Report #7.
[259] Ibid.
[260] Silent Spring Revisited, Chapter 10, 159-74.

<u>Changes Everything</u>.[261] Klein's focus is on the urgent need to deal with the fact of climate change and its troubling consequences. As she develops her argument, Klein observes that whenever the driving forces of capitalism are threatened, the corporations will make the plea, one way or another, that those pressing for change are really one of more of the following ilk:

Communists, or Socialists, or Anti-economic growth and development, or all the foregoing.

Kohn moves from his negative view of the modern environmental movement to claiming "it is now believed…that 'at least 80% of all cancers are caused by synthetic chemicals'… This perception now pervades all strata of US society."[262] According to Kohn, this widespread perception is a distorted one – a perception at odds with reality. Yet, he provides no source for his quotation, and no development of its disproof other than his unsupported assertion that it has been disproved.

At the end of Kohn's otherwise well-written piece his "disclaimers" absolve his employers and others of any responsibility for his expressed views. It is not a far-fetched assumption to believe that neither his "current employer (Zoecon Corporation)," nor his "erstwhile employer (Chevron Chemical Company)", or "the National Agricultural Chemical Association…,"[263] would have any problem whatsoever with his observations and conclusions.

Furthermore, it is fair to surmise that none of the following would have any objection to C.F. Wilkinson's staunch defense of chemicals in his piece entitled, "Being More Realistic About Chemical Carcinogenesis."[264]:

- The National Food Processors Association
- The Tobacco Industry
- Juvenon (a biotechnology company)
- The Texaco Foundation
- Chemagro
- Monsanto Corp.

---

[261] Naomi Klein, <u>This Changes Everything: Capitalism vs. The Climate </u>(NY: Simon & Schuster, 2014).
[262] Ibid, 170.
[263] Ibid, 173.
[264] Chris F. Wilkinson, "Being More Realistic About Chemical Carcinogenesis," www.pmep.cce.cornell.edu/facts-slides-self/facts/gen-pubre-carcin-wilkinson.

- Stauffer Chemicals
- Burdock & Associates
- Dow AgroSciences
- NuFarm Inc.
- Proctor & Gambles
- Agro-Gov S.A.
- Council for LAS/LAB Environmental Research
- The California Canners & Growers Association
- Novartis Corporation
- The Chemical Manufacturers Association
- The Flavor Extract Manufacturers Association

Why could we expect the above companies/organizations to look favorably upon the Wilkinson thesis? Simply put, they have at one time or another provided financial backing for 28 percent of Wilkinson's cited sources.[265]

Whether it is collusion or complicity, (or happenstance?), one cannot be certain, but in the last 10-15 years there has been a growing effort to discredit the toxicological analyses of cancer's causal links to pesticides. Increasingly, articles on the matter highlight the virtues of the epidemiological studies, as well as bolder and bolder cries for the Federal Government to permit the direct testing of pesticides on human beings.

Up to now, epidemiological studies of pesticide impact on human beings have, by necessity, relied upon studies of people known to have been exposed to pesticide poisoning due to such things as accidents and spillages at pesticide production plants, pesticide distribution facilities, or as pesticide applicators. In addition, epidemiologists have been able to study folks who were likely to have been exposed because of their occupation such as

---

[265] As determined by scanning Wilkinson's cited experts, i.e., his 29 cited sources and 51 footnotes through the Integrity of Science database which identifies the nature of "Non-profit Organizations Receiving Corporate Funding." Integrity of Science is a Center for Science in the Public Interest (CSPI) Project which seeks to:
1. Promote "full disclosure of conflicts of interest during the federal advisory appointment process, in academic journals, and in the media," and
2. Challenge conflicts of interest and "undue influence by corporate funded and/or questionable science…" (www.cspinet.org)

farmers, farm families, and those who routinely work with pesticides. The chemical companies seem to hold to a certain degree of confidence that if humans were used as guinea pigs, the lab results would at least support a higher level of acceptable risk – and consequent higher levels of sales and profits.

In fact, chemical companies have been quietly funding "clinical studies that expose paid volunteers to pesticides and then submitting the data to the EPA to persuade regulators not to further restrict applications of the widely used chemicals."[266]

The George W. Bush administration had placed a temporary ban on the practice of using "human guinea pigs" by asking the National Academy of Sciences to review what the chemical companies have been doing from scientific and ethical viewpoints.

However, the EPA planned to spend $7 million along with $2 million provided by the American Chemical Council "to pay poor families to continue to use pesticides in their homes." The intent included offering the families "$970 each, as well as a camcorder and children's clothing to … serve as guinea pigs for the study."[267] The "human guinea pigs" would be used, in the fullest sense of the word, to determine the impact of pesticides on human health.

In June 2005, a special Congressional report on "Human Pesticide Experiments"[268] noted that among other things:

- The EPA intended "to review over 20 studies that intentionally dosed human subjects with pesticides."
- The "pesticides administered…include 'highly hazardous' poisons, suspected carcinogens, and suspected neurotoxicants."
- "The studies…appear to routinely violate ethical standards."

---

[266] "Pesticide tests on humans banned," Omaha World Herald (December 16, 2001), 10A.

[267] "Bill Moyers' speech on receiving Harvard Med's Global Environment Citizen Award," Crestone Eagle, January 2005, 27.

[268] Human Pesticide Experiments, prepared by the U.S. House of Representative's Committee on Government Reform-Minority Staff, Special Investigations Division, and Senator Barbara Boxer's Environmental Staff, prepared at Senator Boxer's and Representative Henry A. Waxman's request.

- In 22 of the 24 studies submitted to the EPA, the Boxer-Waxman report notes that there were "significant and widespread deficiencies" which were "in violation of ethical standards, the experiments appear to have inflicted harm on human subjects, failed to obtain informed consent, diminished adverse outcomes, and lacked scientific validity." (p.1)
- "Nearly one-third of the studies reviewed were specifically designed to cause harm to the human test subjects or to put them at risk of harm." (p,10)
- "…few, if any of the 22 studies appear to have a large enough Sample size to have adequate statistical power. /for example, three off the experiments involved just six subjects each. One study was conducted on a single subject." (p.23)
- The 22 studies exhibited a "Systematic Dismissal of Adverse Events" (pp.23-25) as well s a "Failure to Conduct Long-Term Medical Follow-up." (pp. 26-27)

The chemical companies' clinical studies of human health response to being intentionally exposed to pesticides are a "slippery slope" ethically and morally. Just because a Panel composed of the Institute of Medicine of the National Academy of Sciences has recommended a broadening of permissible human biomedical tests in prisons does not make the slippery slope any less slippery.[269]

Yes, the subjects in the study may agree o the tests. Yes, they are paid for their participation. However, are those human guinea pigs exposed to pesticides through ingestion or inhaling, drinking or eating, informed they are receiving the real thing as opposed to the other subjects in the double-blind tests who would receive only a placebo? If they are not so informed, those people are going to be betting on the chance of avoiding being exposed to the real thing and its detrimental impact upon their health. Indeed, are they informed about what those detriment might be? Are there safeguards in place to assure understanding?

---

[269] Ian Urbina, "Panel Suggests Using Inmates in Drug Trial," NY Times (August 13, 2006).

On the latter point, there is an immense ethical issue: Non-compliance with the principle of informed consent. If they are so informed, the companies' studies may conform to a certain level of ethical practice, but scientific validity would be in serious jeopardy. The chemical companies and scientists would be caught in a double bind with or without double-blinded research designs.

However, the chemical companies do have access to more direct influence regarding legalization of distribution and use of their products. On January 15, 2004, Earthjustice filed a lawsuit against the EPA on behalf of a coalition of environmental organizations. This lawsuit sought to "stop the EPA from giving illegal special access to a group of chemical organizations."[270]

It is no secret that the chemical companies have played a major role in funding studies that somehow reflect favorably upon the industry and its products. It is also no deep secret that the chemical companies court favors with state, local, and national regulatory agencies.

Indeed, as the President's Cancer Panel contends, "U.S. regulation of environmental contaminants is rendered ineffective by…undue industry influence."[271] It is just that when the open secrets hit the headlines, the collusion between government and industry becomes raw and potentially devastating to the "Whistleblowers" such as Dr. Omar Shafey:

---

[270] "EPA Sued for Illegally Taking Direction from Chemical Industry Group," (Beyond Pesticides, January 20, 2004). www.earthjustice.org/news/documents/104/FIFRAComplaint.pdf%20.
[271] PCP 2010, ii.

Speaking Truth to Power: Pesticide Wars & The Troubling Story of Dr. Omar Shafey[272]

*In February 1998, the Florida Department of Health (FDOH) hired Dr. Shafey to track pesticide-related health problems. Although pesticide usage in Florida is comparatively high, cases of pesticide poisoning have been woefully underreported there for years.... After being hired ... (*Shafey*) uncovered previously unrecognized pesticide exposure routes ... Initially Shafey's hard work paid off. He was honored with appreciation awards by state and county health departments ... And he earned the respect of diverse communities: colleagues, academics, farm workers, and ordinary citizens ... Yet two years after Shafey began his job, he was fired and forcibly removed from his office in Tallahassee after allegedly overcharging his department $12.50 on a travel reimbursement claim.*

Shafey claims he was harassed and ultimately sacked for resisting pressure from his supervisors to present results more pleasing to powerful agriculture interests. He is suing the Florida health department and two of his former bosses for wrongful dismissal under whistleblower statutes as well as for infringement of his First Amendment rights....

Shafey's star began its meteoric descent after he refused to alter his recommendations against spraying areas with Malathion to control agricultural pest(s).... After analyzing medical reports and interviewing patients, Shafey concluded the spraying was making people sick... Florida deployed Malathion against an outbreak of Mediterranean fruit fly, or med fly...

By October 1998 Shafey had confirmed 123 cases of illness relate to the spraying, a finding that was later published in the U.S. Center for disease Control and Prevention's Morbidity & Mortality Weekly Report. The same month Shafey wrote the report...the final med fly report FDOH issued was stripped of both Shafey's recommendation and his name. Shafey says he was pressured for months by his supervisors to change his recommendation and

---

[272] Excerpted with permission from "Pesticide Wars – The Troubling Story of Dr. Omar Shafey," by Karen Charman www.pmac.net/pesticide_wars; originally published at www.tompaine.com/features/2001/11/16/index. Best accessed currently at www.karencharman.com, or at http://www.mindfully.org/pesticides/fired. Accessed February 3, 2016.

conform to health department policy that was much less aggressive about documenting cases of pesticide poisoning than he was.

In early December 1999, he says his boss...suggested Shafey consider money and politics as driving forces behind the way the department treated health issues involving pesticides, and that if Shafey could not "bend" to accommodate FDOH policy, he should leave.

NOTE: In light of the furor generated by Shafey's 1998 report, it is worth noting Watts & Williamson's "Snapshot" below:

Table 5

A Snapshot of Recent Field Surveys of Pesticide Poisoning

Bangladesh, 2014 –85% of applicators reported suffering gastrointestinal problems during and after spraying, 63% eye problems, 61 % skin problems, and 47% physical weakness. Most commonly used pesticides: Ops (organic phosphates) and synthetic pyrethroids.

India, 2014 – a survey by the Calcutta School of Tropical Medicine and the NRS Medical College found that 30% of farmers using pesticides in a district in West Bengal were experiencing neurological symptoms. In 2012 a survey of pesticide-exposed farmers in Punjab, India, reported 94.4% exhibited some symptoms of poisoning.

Burkina Faso, 2013 – 82.66% of farmers surveyed reported having experienced at least one ailment during or just after spraying, most commonly central nervous system effects. Of the cases reported to a health care centre, 53% were unintentional ingestion, 28% suicides ,and 19% occupational use.

Pakistan, 2012 – in a small study of female workers picking cotton 3-15 days after pesticides were last used, 100% of them experienced headache, nausea and vomiting.

South Korea, 2012 – acute occupational pesticide poisoning amongst young male Korean farmers was reported to be 24.7%.

Brazil, 2012 – in a small survey in Brazil, 44.8% of rural workers involved in vegetable production reported health problems whilst using pesticides. A survey of workers involved in potato production reported that 33% of them had experienced intoxication at least once.

Iran, 2012 – 12% of pesticide applicators involved in rice growing suffer acute pesticide poisoning.

Sudan, 2011 – a study reported 27% poisoning rate among small vegetable farmers.

Colombia, 2012 – the Public Health Surveillance System reported 6,650 poisoning cases from use of pesticides in 2008, increasing to 7,405 in 2009 and 8,016 in 2010, most commonly caused by OP and carbamate insecticides.

SOURCE: Watts & Williamson, 19, Box 1.2

On November 1, 2001 a court ruling held that Shafey's case could move forward. However, he ultimately lost his case. Not because of any court filings regarding the content and substance of his research, but on legal technicalities. In fact, the above "Snapshot" highlights how it is that Shafey's 1998 findings continue to be underscored around the globe. All of the 11 surveys cited by Watts & Williamson between 2011-2014; and every one of these surveys proclaim the bitter truth and warnings conveyed by Dr. Oma Shafey 13-16 years before.

The Shafey incident points out how influential the chemical industry is in the Florida state agency charged with regulating the use of the industry's products. Mary DeVany, chair of the American Industrial Hygiene Association's Social Concerns Committee, claims:

> *There's a lot of pressure being put on people to modify, soften their tone, or hedge their reports to say something is possible instead of 'here's the evidence that it happened'... We're talking about an increased acceptance of unethical behavior – about supervisors and managers putting pressure on their technical professionals to perform unethical acts.*[273]

Dr. Shafey has subsequently worked for the American Cancer Society in Atlanta, Georgia, the Emory University's Rollins School of Public Health. He has recently moved to Abu Dhabi, where he is Senior Officer for Medical Research for the Ministry of Health, United Arab Emirates.

The question is how many other Dr. Omar Shafeys are there across the country and the world who have been silenced? How many have given up the fight? How much evidence is being withheld which would otherwise help convict pesticides, pesticide applicators, pesticide distributors and pesticide manufacturers of public health crimes? The fate of Omar Shafey strongly suggests there is much that is being hidden – and suppressed. And, the problem is not going

---

[273] Charman.

away. It is getting bigger and more ominous by the day, ever since January 20, 2017. Stay tuned. (See pages 214-219).

■■■

The Case of Dr. Melvin Dwayne Reuber[274]

From 1958 to 1980, Dr. Reuber established a reputation as a conscientious expert in cancer research authoring over 130 journal articles and in 1980 receiving an outstanding rating at the Frederick (Maryland) Cancer Research /center (FCRC) as director of the Experimental Pathology Laboratory. One year later Reuber was in trouble and has never found employment since then that has been commensurate with his qualifications and experience. What happened?

In the mid-1970s, Reuber's work involved assessing the impact of a variety of chemicals upon experimental animals. As he examined slide-upon-slide of rodent specimens regarding the presence or absence of cancerous tumors, Reuber's diagnoses were often at variance with those of his colleagues. Reuber tended to observe malignancy when others viewed benign tumors. His studies led to the banning of the pesticides aldrin, dieldrin, chlordane and heptachlor. He was highly praised by his supervisor who saw to it that Reuber was granted a $50,000 raise in salary.

Shortly, thereafter Reuber 's research led him to conclude that in 16 of 18 cases he had to disagree with previous rodent studies by the National Cancer Institute where somehow they had "missed cancers that put chemicals in a bad light. Underlying these discrepancies was the possibility of fraud by some chemical industry scientists...[275] However, as things turned out, it was Reuber whose reputation became tainted by accusations of fraud and incompetency.

The same supervisor, who had praised him so highly months before, turned on him and widely published charges that Reuber could never have accomplished the research he claimed to have completed. In addition, Reuber was criticized for using agency

---

[274] Brian Martin, "Critics of pesticides: Whistleblowing or suppression of dissent?" Philosophy and Social Action, Vol.22, No. 3, July - September, 1996.
[275] Ibid, 4-5.

letterhead in his communications with interest groups advocating pesticide regulations.[276] One wonders:

- Would the Frederick Cancer Research Center have really minded if Reuber had commended the use of the same pesticides, using FCRC letterhead to do so?
- What would the last 20 years have been like for Dr. Reuber, if he had just kept his observations to himself? Why couldn't he have just gone along with a system of suppressing the truth?
- What may have been the connection between the FCRC and the Chemical Industry?
- Why, indeed, couldn't Melvin Reuber have kept his mouth shut, and his letter writing at bay? The answer to this rhetorical question is clear. Dr. Reuber needed to live with himself. The same is more than likely true for Dennis Bishop.

The Case of Dennis Bishop, Cooperative Extension Agent

In September 2000, Dennis Bishop, a Stafford County, Virginia, Extension Agent at Virginia Tech (Virginia Polytechnic Institute and State University, Blacksburg, Virginia) was suddenly transferred to a temporary and terminal six-month position. Approximately one month prior to Bishop's reassignment, he had received most positive performance evaluation by his supervisor. What happened?

Two weeks before his unexplained reassignment, Bishop had written a letter to the editor of the Fredericksburg Free Lance-Star responding to a column "bashing organic agriculture,"[277] by Dennis Avery of the Hudson Institute. The American Civil Liberties Union filed suit on Bishop's behalf claiming a violation of free speech, noting he had written the letter "at home, on his own time, on his

---

[276] Ibid, 5-6.
[277] "Ag Extension Agent Fired After Defending Organics," Beyond Pesticides Daily News Archive, February 22, 2001.
www.beyondpesticides.org/NEWS/daily_news_archive/02_22_01.him.

own computer and did not identify himself as an extension employee."[278]

Bishop immediately submitted his 30-day notice to Virginia Tech, took alternative employment for a few months until being hired in April 2001 by the Maryland Cooperative Extension. The settlement with Virginia Tech came to fruition in U.S. District Court in Alexandria, Virginia, on May 25, 2001. Virginia Tech was held by the settlement to pay Bishop $$13,767, and to state, if requested for a job reference regarding Mr. Bishop, "only that he quit his post and make no reference to the letter nor suggest that his job performance was unsatisfactory."[279]

Dennis Bishop's experience has all the earmarks of an employer attempting to suppress a dissident and the dissident's views from reaching the public realm. Is it due to fear that being known to condone such "radical" views that Virginia Tech would lose funding support from critical donors? After all, Bishop had not just defended organic farming, he claimed farming techniques employing the usage of pesticides "rape the earth."[280]

Dr. Omar Shafey, Dr. Melvin Reuber, and Dennis Bishop are but a few of the known cases of those who have questioned the safety of pesticides and lost their jobs for saying so. Rachel Carson knew what the forces of suppression were like,[281] as did Robert Rudd who wrote a successful book,[282] but lost his job. Robert Rudd: one more victim of corporate power.

---

[278] Pamela Gould, "Ex-agent, Tech settle suit: School agrees to pay Bishop $13,767," Fredericksburg Free Lance-Star, June 5, 2001. www.fredericksburg.com/NEWS/FLSS/2001/062001/302083.

[279] Ibid, 1.

[280] Ibid.

[281] See Souder for an extensive description of the corporate pressures, propaganda, and character attacks on Rachel Carson after the publication of Silent Spring.

[282] Robert Rudd, Pesticides and the Living Landscape (Madison: The University of Wisconsin Press, 1964).

The Case of Robert Rudd

In 1965 Roland Clement, a staff biologist with the National Audubon Society, reviewed Robert Rudd's book, noting that Rudd "is one of the pioneer students of the effects of the new chemical pesticides in the landscape."[283] Clement points out that Rudd and Genelly had published on the subject nearly 10 years before in 1956.[284] In other words, Rudd's earlier study was published six years prior to Rachel Carson's Silent Spring (1962).

Clement concludes that Rudd's thesis as per our option in dealing with agriculture-related pests comes down to two choices:

- *To work with nature in keeping pest populations under control, or*
- *To press for an increasingly synthetic landscape, where man takes on the task, and the risks, of keeping all factors in balance.*[285]

While Clement sees Rudd as "conservative, calm, and generous in his appraisals," he experiences Rudd's book as a:

...clear indictment of the eradication philosophy of the control entomologists and of the predator control work of the past two decades that, in the name of science, overlooked or disregarded basic ecology and must therefore be labeled cosmic thinking.[286]

Rudd's book was ready to be published long before Carson's best seller. He had every reason to believe that the Conservation Foundation was set to have it published.

---

[283] Roland C. Clement, "Pesticides and the Living Landscape," Natural Resources Journal, October 1965, 432-434. http://lawschool.unm.edu/nrj/volumes/05/2/15_clement-pesticides.pdf. Accessed March,10,2015.

[284] Rudd & Genelly, *Pesticides: Their Use and Toxicity in Relation to Wildlife* (California Department of Fish and Game 1956).

[285] Clement, 432.

[286] Ibid, 433.

However, "(T)he corporate publisher to which the Conservation Foundation gave the manuscript turned it down as a 'polemic.'" Ultimately, the University of Wisconsin Press published the manuscript, having been read by over 200 scientists, "but Rudd lost a promotion at the University of California at Davis and his career was threatened. He was dismissed without notice or cause in 1964 from his position at the University's Agricultural E Experiment Station."[287]

The Shafey, Reuber, Bishop, and Rudd cases are but tiny molecules on the tip of the iceberg that attempts to freeze debate. However, one of the most effective approaches to freezing debate is to place the facts at the very bottom of the iceberg.

The Case of the Syngenta Chemical Company

The Natural Resource Defense Council (NRDC) alerted the EPA of two studies indicating atrazine's causal association with sexual deformities in frogs and prostate cancer in workers manufacturing the chemical. NRDC and others suspect "Syngenta may have illegally suppressed these findings." EPA ruled in June 2000 that atrazine is "not likely" to be a human carcinogen, but EPA was not aware at the time of the studies alluded to here – studies that may have been purposely withheld from EPA by Syngenta.[288]

---

[287] John Bellamy Foster and Bret Clark, "Rachel Carson's Ecological Critique," Monthly Review (February 2008, Volume 59, Issue 09). http://monthlyreview.org/2008/02/01/rachel-carson-ecological-critique. 6.
[288] "Two New Studies Reveal Dangers of Atrazine," Beyond Pesticides Daily News Archive, July 2, 2002. www.beyondpesticides.org/NEWS/daily_news_archive/07_02_02.htm As of February 2010, for the seven states highlighted in this book, the number of atrazine-based pesticides registered ranged from two (2) in Kansas to 136 in Florida. (Source: National Pesticide Retrieval System at www.ppis.ceris.purdue.edu/npublic). **NOTE: As of March 8, 2016, this site was no longer available (re-affirmed as unavailable on August 25, 2018). The site allegedly replacing it (www.stte.ceris.purdue.edu) does not list the number of**

One the other hand, there appears to be at least one case where EPA withheld critical information, despite Syngenta's "careful" reporting. In August 2009, the Huffington Post reported that:

One of the nation's most widely-used herbicides has been found to exceed federal safety limits in drinking water in four states, but water customers have not been told and the Environmental Protection Agency has not published the results.[289]

Investigative reporter Danielle Ivory notes:

The yearly average levels of atrazine in drinking water violated the federal standard at least ten times in communities in Illinois, Indiana, Ohio, and Kansas... In addition, more than 40 water systems in those states showed spikes in atrazine levels that normally would have triggered automatic notification of customers. In none of those case were residents alerted.[290]

Of course, both the EPA and Syngenta responded that since atrazine has been declared by EPA as posing "no threat to the safety of our drinking water supplies" there is no need for concern. This is an entirely different take on the issue than that of the European Union. "In 2004, the EU banned atrazine because it was consistently showing up in drinking water and health officials, aware of ongoing studies, said they could not find sufficient

---

pesticides registered in each state. The only way to find that out is to go through the laborious process of typing in the name of each pesticide, and then tallying up the score. This writer decided he had better things to do! The point is this: For whatever reason, from February 2010, it has become much more difficult to obtain critical information concerning the extent of pesticide use in the United States.

[289] Danielle Ivory, "EPA Fails to Inform Public About Weed-Killer in Drinking Water," Huffington Post, August 3, 2009. www.huffingtonpost.com/2009/08/23/epa-fails-to-inform-publi_n_26686, 1.

[290] Ibid.

evidence the chemical is safe."[291] The EU's policy stance on this issue adheres to the Precautionary Principle (See Chapter 10).

In 2003, the EPA and Syngenta reached an agreement that EPA would approve the use of atrazine as long as Syngenta would agree to pay for the weekly monitoring of 150 watersheds, testing for levels of atrazine. Instead of transparency being a product of this government-corporate deal, we find only apparent collusion and deception. For example, the Huffington Post reports hat in the case of quarterly reports, the citizens of Mt. Olive, Illinois, "were told that the highest level of atrazine in their drinking water (in 2008) was 2ppb. However, the EPA data shows a spike in June of 16.47ppb."[292]

When asked why the EPA did not publish this data provided by Syngenta to the EPA, the justification appears to come in dual terms:

1. The Safe Water Drinking Water Act only requires cities to report state collected data, thus legally speaking the data provided by Syngenta can be ignored,
2. The EPA administrator claimed the data was readily available on EPA's website.

Danielle Ivory discovered that the desired data was "one of the only items on the docket not posted on the website, Instead, the data is listed as available ONLY through the Freedom of Information Act.[293]

Perhaps Nicholas D. Kristof best describes the issue we face in his NY Times piece, "The Cancer Lobby: Who knew that carcinogens had their own lobby in Washington?"[294] when he says:

---

[291] Ibid, 2.

[292] Ibid, 3.

[293] Ibid.

[294] Nicholas D. Kristof, "The Cancer Lobby: Who knew that carcinogens had their own lobby in Washington?" The NY Times (October 6, 2012) www.nytimes.com/2012/10/07/opinion/Sunday/kristof-the-cancer-lobby.

The larger issue is whether the federal government should be a watchdog for public health, or a lap dog for industry.

The Case of USEPA Expert Panelist Michelle Boone

Journalist Zoe Schlanger reports the experience of an expert recruited by the USEPA to serve on EPA's Scientific Advisory Panel for Pesticide Regulation. Schlanger notes that at an EPA panel meeting in the Spring of 2012, Miami University of Ohio Ecologist Michelle Boone was aghast that the EPA had "disqualified from rule-making all but one study on the effect of atrazine on amphibians. The lone remaining study was funded by Syngenta, the manufacturer of atrazine. Most other papers on atrazine had found some connection between the chemical and adverse effects on amphibians. The Syngenta-funded study showed none."[295]

To Michelle Boone, it was more than obvious that given Syngenta's financial stake in maintaining atrazine on EPA's approved list of "Safe" chemicals, there was an equally obvious conflict of interest at work, especially given the "paperwork she and her colleague were required to file certifying that *they* (emphasis added) presented no conflict of interest by serving on the panel, this seemed patently bizarre."[296]

Rather than playing along and pretending nothing is amiss with the EPA process, Boone mobilized a nationwide group of ecotoxicologists to critique EPA's rule-making protocols on all chemicals, not just atrazine. Schlanger observes from the Boone Report, that the EPA, in collaboration with the chemical industry establishes the methodological guidelines for chemical studies. The end result, normally, is that the chemical industry is the "only entity that can afford to conduct the research to the USEPA's specifications... Therefore, all or most of the data used in risk assessments may come from industry-supplied research, despite clear conflicts of interest..."[297]

---

[295] Zoe Schlanger, "Does the EPA Favor Industry When Assessing Chemical Dangers?" Newsweek (September 5, 2014. www.newsweek.com/does-epa-favor-industry-when-assessing-chemical-dangers-268168. Accessed June 6, 2015.
[296] Ibid.
[297] Ibid.

Let us consider, in more detail, the Boone Report[298] as developed by Boone and her team of 14 other scientists:

- This is not a diatribe directed at the USEPA. Note for example, the preface statement:

We… offer solutions to improve the risk assessment process which would reduce the potential for and perception of bias in a process that is crucial for environment and human health.[299]

- But of course, it is not uncritical, as warned two sentences later:

The ongoing reassessment of atrazine's impact on amphibians underscores some to the pitfalls of the USEPA's current approach and illustrates how the USEPA's directive to protect human and environmental health may be undermined.

- Under the heading of "Concerns with the USEPA's risk assessment process," Boone and Associates postulate that:
  + COI's (Conflicts of Interest) "are currently ingrained in the process…"[300]

    Indeed, COI's and industry bias appears to be "hardwired" in the EPA pesticide risk process.

Therefore, the Boone Report claims that among other things, the EPA should:

- Amend its severely limiting criteria that effectively eliminates any study that is NOT sponsored by the chemical industry.
- Rely more on field studies, rather than on laboratory research.
- Be much more transparent regarding the Scientific Advisory Panel's recommendations.
- "Adopt the scientific 'weight-of-evidence' approach to reaching conclusions regarding the safety of chemicals….

---

[298] Michelle D. Boone, et al, "Pesticide Regulation amid the Influence of Industry," Bioscience (October 2014, Vol 64, No. 10), 917-922) http://bioscience.oxfordjournals.org.

[299] Boone, 917.

[300] Boone, 918-920.

- "Exercise precaution rather than the 'innocent until proven guilty' approach to pesticide regulation."[301]

The Case Made by the Chemical Industry

The Chemical Manufacturers Association (CMA) has found a convenient whipping boy/strawman designed to divert attention from the issues and research concerning the potential carcinogenic effect of the products manufactured by the 175-member companies. By attacking the emerging field of environmental medicine, perhaps any charges concerning carcinogens in the environment can easily be discounted as quackery. Witness the CMA's statements on the matter.

NOTE: What follows is taken in-directly from CMA's website by Get Set, Inc, and is presented here with permission on February 9, 2016 by Steve Tvedten, editor, who cites CMA's "Fair Use Notice" as justification for placing the information below in the public realm.[302]

- *For many patients, environmental illness has become the explanation for a combination of symptoms for which they've found no other acceptable explanation.*
- *Environmental medicine specialists believe their patients are severely 'allergic' to the world they live in o the extent that many of them cannot function in society.*
- *Environmental illness patients generally lead troubled lives and have genuine problems coping with family, work and life-style pressures. They often eagerly accept environmental illness as the explanation for their condition and undertake the costly life-style changes including moving to new environments and eliminating all synthetic agents from their homes that are part of treatment.[303]*

---

[301] Boone, 920-921.

[302] "The Chemical Manufacturers Association's Environmental Illness Briefing Paper," 1990. www.getipm.com/articles/CMA-briefing.html.

[303] Ibid, 1.

- *The label of environmental illness is a misdiagnosis and condemns these patients to the life of an outcast with little hope of cure. It is essential that their described symptoms be taken seriously. These patients deserve the best medical evaluation and treatment consistent with established medical principles.*
- *It is not the legitimacy of the patients that is in question, but the alleged environmental cause. Failure to recognize this critical difference can result in enormous costs to the patient, to industry and to society.[304]*
- *The concept of multiple chemical hypersensitivities as a disease entity in which the patient experiences numerous symptoms from numerous chemicals and foods caused by disturbance of the immune system lacks scientific foundation. Published reports off such cases are anecdotal and without proper controls… As defined and presented by its proponents, multiple chemical hypersensitivities constitute a belief and not a disease…. Some of the patients who believe they have environmental illness also have symptoms characteristic of psychosomatic illness.[305]*

The gist of CMA's argument, then, is that environmental medicine is an illegitimate field of medical science and practice, chemical sensitivity is a hoax, and those folks so diagnosed with MCS are hypochondriacs and social misfits. Therefore, any claim that chemicals in the environment can cause serious public illness is a hoax. Case dismissed!

"Chemophobia" and controversy being the "work product of an environmentalist," appears to be the worldview of those "researchers" and lobbyists funded by the chemical manufacturers.[306] It is the belief system that most likely allows "the purveyors of products and chemicals, and legislators, regulators, and scientists reluctant to bite the money-laden hands that feed them"[307] to sleep at night.

---

[304] Ibid, 2.
[305] Ibid, 5.
[306] Sherman, ix.
[307] Ibid, 2.

On the other hand, the chemical companies, such as Novartis, have been known to try having it both ways. In November 1990 Sandoz (now Novartis) was scheduled to present anti-MCS information" at a medical conference in San Francisco where they were prepared to make the claim that people with MCS are simply "mentally ill." While such a claim would help undermine the whole notion of pesticides being the culprit and cause of anything like MCS and take Novartis' production of these chemicals off the hook, labeling MCS as a psychiatric condition would set Novartis' production of psychiatric drugs in a favorable marketing position.[308]

In July 1997, a World Conference on Breast Cancer, sponsored by the World Conference on Breast Cancer Foundation (WCBCF),[309] was held in Kingston, Ontario, Canada, the site of the second highest incidence of breast cancer in North America. At this conference on the banks of Lake Ontario (the catchment of pollutants from the other Great Lakes, their tributaries, chemical run-off from farms, waste from factories, chemical run-ff from farms, waste from factories, sewage and road run-off, to name a few), the Conference had a few things to say about the "Collective Cancer Establishment." It is, they proclaimed, as complicit with "mainstream science as the emperor's tailors."[310]

The Collective Cancer Establishment at that time was believed to be composed of the National Cancer Institute, the National Institute for Health, the funds-receiving research universities, the American Cancer Society, and the Chemical-Pharmaceutical-Biotech Industry.[311]

Perhaps all that has been said in this chapter comes down to saying the fox appears to be guarding the henhouse. Si Kahn and Elizabeth Minnich put forth the claim that the merging of corporate

---

[308] Ann McCampbell, M.D., "Multiple Chemical Sensitivities Under Siege," www.getipm.com/personal/mcs-campbell.

[309] The WCBCF is "governed by a voluntary Board of Directors made up of breast cancer survivors, grass roots conference volunteers, aboriginal representatives, researchers, clinician, corporate sponsor representatives, and others knowledgeable in breast cancer issues." www.wcbcf.ca/foundation/profile.

[310] Sherman, 217-218. See also: Samuel Epstein, The Politics of Cancer Revisited (East Ridge Press, 1998, xvi).

[311] See Samuel S. Epstein's biting critique of the American Cancer Society as "The World's Wealthiest 'Nonprofit' Institution," in Cancer-Gate: How to Win the Losing Cancer War(Baywood Publishing Company, 2005, 79-92).

power with government services such as prisons, tramples individual freedoms.[312] Could we add to that the trampling of human life and truth itself?

The Trampling of Human Life and Truth:
The Case of Dr. Tyrone Hayes,
Professor of Integrative Biology, UC Berkeley

In her New Yorker[313] piece of February 2014, Rachel Aviv reports:

Hundreds of Syngenta's memos, notes, and e-mails have been unsealed following the settlement, in 2012, of two class-action suits brought by twenty-three Midwestern cities and towns that accused Syngenta of 'concealing atrazine's true dangerous nature' and contaminating their drinking water. Stephen Tillery, the lawyer who argued the cases, said, 'Tyrone's work gave us the scientific basis for the lawsuit.'

Hayes has devoted the past fifteen years to studying atrazine, and during that time scientists around the world have expanded on his findings, suggesting that the herbicide is associated with birth defects in humans as well as in animals. The company documents show that while Hayes was studying atrazine, Syngenta was studying him, as he had long expected. Syngenta's public-relations team had drafted a list of four goals. The first was 'discredit Hayes.' In a spiral-bound notebook, Syngenta's communications manager, Sherry Ford...wrote that... 'If TH is involved in scandal, enviros will drop him... What's motivating Hayes? --- basic question.

In 1994, the EPA, expressing concerns about atrazine's health effects, announced that it would start a scientific review. Syngenta assembled a panel of scientists and professors, through a consulting firm called EcoRisk, to study the herbicide. Hayes eventually joined the group. His first experiment showed that male tadpoles exposed to atrazine developed less muscle surrounding their vocal cords, and he hypothesized that the chemical had the

---

[312] Si Kahn and Elizabeth Minnich, The Fox in the Henhouse: How Privatization Threatens Democracy (Berrett-Koehler Publishers, 2005).

[313] Rachel Aviv, "A Valuable Reputation: After Tyrone Hayes said that a chemical was harmful, its maker pursued him," The New Yorker, February 10, 2014. www.newyorker.com/magazine/2014/02/10/a-valuable-reputation, Accessed February 11, 2015. Excerpted and quoted here with permission.

potential to reduce testosterone levels. 'I have been losing lots of sleep over this,' he wrote one of EcoRisk panel member, in the summer of 2000. 'I realize the implications and of course want to make sure that everything possible has been done and controlled for."

After a conference call, he was surprised by the way the company kept critiquing what seemed to be trivial aspects of the work... He decided to resign from the panel, (saying in part) If I continue... It will appear to my colleagues that I have been part of a plan to bury important data.'

Hayes repeated the experiments using funds from Berkeley and the National Science foundation. Afterward, he wrote top the panel, 'Although I do not want to make a big deal out of it until I have all of the data analyzed and decoded – I feel I should warn you that I think something very strange is coming up in these animals.' After dissecting the frogs, he noticed that some could not be clearly identified as male or female: they had both testes and ovaries. Others had multiple testes that were deformed.

In January 2001, Syngenta...asked to meet with him privately, but Hayes insisted on the presence of his students, a few colleagues, and his wife... Syngenta introduced a guest speaker, a statistical consultant, who listed numerous errors in Hayes's report and concluded that the results were not statistically significant. Hayes's wife, Katherine Kim, said that the consultant seemed to be trying to 'make Tyrone look as foolish as possible....'

Hayes later e-mailed three of the scientists, telling them, 'I was insulted, felt railroaded and, in fact, felt that some dishonest and unethical activity was going on.' When he explained what had happened to Theo Colburn, the scientist who had popularized the theory that industrial chemicals could alter hormones, she advised him, 'Don't go home the same way twice.' Colburn was convinced that her office had been bugged, and that industry representatives followed her. She told Hayes to 'keep looking over your shoulder' and to be careful whom he let in his lab. She warned him, 'You have got to protect yourself.'

Hayes published his atrazine work in the Proceedings of the National Academy of Sciences a year and a half after quitting the panel. He wrote that what he called 'hermaphroditism' was induced in frogs by exposure to atrazine at levels thirty times below what the E.P.A. permits in water. He hypothesized that the chemical could be a factor in the decline in amphibian populations, a phenomenon observed all over the world. In an e-mail sent the day before the publication, he congratulated the students in his lab for taking the 'ethical stance' by continuing the work on their own. 'We (and our principles) have been tested, and I believe we have not only passed but exceeded expectations,' he wrote. 'Science is a principle and a process of seeking truth. Truth cannot be purchased and, thus, truth cannot be altered by money. Professorship is not a career, but rather a life's pursuit. The people with whom I work daily exemplify and remind me of this promise.'

. . .

According to company e-mails, Syngenta was distressed by Hayes's work. Its public-relations team compiled a database of more than a hundred 'supportive third party stakeholders,' including twenty-five professors, who could defend atrazine or act as "spokespeople on Hayes.' The P.R. team suggested that the company 'purchase Tyrone Hayes as a search word on the internet, so that any time someone searches for Tyrone's material, the first thing they see is our material.' The proposal was later expanded to include the phrases 'amphibian hayes,' 'atrazine frogs,' and 'frog feminization.' (Searching online for "Tyrone Hayes" now brings up an advertisement that says, 'Tyrone Hayes Not Credible.')[314]

. . . .

In early 2003, Hayes was considered for a job at the Nicholas School of the Environment, at Duke. He visited the campus three times, and the university arranged for a real-estate agent to show him and his wife potential homes. When Syngenta learned that Hayes might be moving to North Carolina, where its crop-protection headquarters are situated, Gary Dickson—the company's vice-president of global risk assessment, who a year earlier had established a fifty-thousand-dollar endowment, funded by Syngenta, at the Nicholas School—contacted a dean at Duke. According to documents unsealed in the class-action lawsuits, Dickinson informed the dean of the 'state of the relationship between Dr. Hayes and Syngenta. The company 'wanted to protect our reputation in our community and among our employees'....

---

[314] As of August 28, 2018, this ad no longer appears.

In June 2003, Hayes paid his own way to Washington so that he could present his work at an E.P.A. hearing on atrazine. The agency had evaluated seventeen studies... The E.P.A. found that all seventeen atrazine studies, including Hayes's suffered methodological flaws—contamination of controls, variability in measurement end points, poor animal husbandry—and asked Syngenta to fund a comprehensive experiment that would produce more definitive results. Darcy Kelley, a member of the E.P.A.'s scientific advisory panel and a biology professor at Columbia, said that, at the time, 'I did not think the E.P.A. made the right decision.' The studies by Syngenta scientists had flaws that 'really cast into doubt their ability to carry out their experiments. They couldn't replicate effects that are as easy as falling off a log.' She thought that Hayes's experiments were more respectable, but she wasn't persuaded by Hayes's explanation of the biological mechanism causing deformities.

The E.P.A. approved the continued use of atrazine in October, the same month that the European Commission chose to remove it from the market. The European Union generally takes a precautionary approach to environmental risks, choosing restraint in the face of uncertainty. In the U.S., lingering scientific questions justify delays in regulatory decisions. Since the mid-seventies, the E.P.A. has issued regulations restricting the use of only five industrial chemicals out of more than eighty thousand in the environment....

Syngenta began holding weekly 'atrazine meetings' after the first class-action suit was filed, in 2004. The meetings were attended by toxicologists, the company's counsel, communications staff, and the head of regulatory affairs. To dampen negative publicity from the lawsuit, the group discussed how it could invalidate Hayes's research. (Sherry) *Ford* (Syngenta's Director of Communications, and convener of these meetings) *documented peculiar things he had done ('kept coat on') or phrases he had used ('Is this line clean?').*

'If TH wanted to win the day, and he had the goods,' she wrote, 'he would have produced them when asked.' She noted that Hayes was 'getting in too deep w/enviros,' and searched for ways to get him to 'show his true colors.'

In 2005, Ford made a long list of methods for discrediting him: 'have his work audited by 3rd party,' 'ask journals to retract,' 'set trap to entice him to sue,' 'investigate funding,' 'investigate wife.' The initials of different employees were written in the margins beside entries, presumably because they had been assigned to look into the task. Another set of ideas, discussed at several meetings, was to conduct 'systematic rebuttals of all TH appearances.' One of the company's communications consultants said in an e-mail that she wanted to obtain Hayes's calendar of speaking engagements, so that Syngenta could 'start reaching out to the potential audiences with the Error vs. Truth Sheet,' which would provide 'irrefutable evidence of his polluted messages.' (Syngenta says that many of the documents unsealed in the lawsuits refer to ideas that were never implemented.)

. . . .

(Hayes) began giving more than fifty lectures a year, not just to scientific audiences but to policy institutes, history departments, women's health clinic, food preparers, farmers, and high schools... At his talks, Hayes noticed that one or two men in the audience were dressed, more sharply than the other scientists. They asked questions that seemed to have been designed to embarrass him: Why can't anyone replicate your research? Why won't you share your data? One former student, Ali Stuart, said that 'everywhere Tyrone went there was this guy asking questions that made a mockery of him. We called him the 'Axe Man'....

Syngenta was concerned by Hayes's e-mails and commissioned an outside contractor to do a 'psychological profile' of Hayes. In her notes, Sherry Ford described him as 'bipolar/manic-depressive' and 'paranoid schizo & narcissistic.' Roger Liu, Hayes's student, said that he thought Hayes wrote the e-mails to relieve his anxiety. Hayes often showed the e-mails to his students, who appreciated his rebellious sense of humor. Liu said, 'Tyrone had all these groupies in the lab cheering him on. I was the one in the background saying, you know, 'Man, don't egg them on. Don't poke that beast.'

Syngenta intensified its public-relations campaign in 2009, as it became concerned that activists, touting 'new science' had developed a 'new line of attack.' That year, a paper in Acta Paediatrica, reviewing national records for thirty million births, found that children conceived between April and July, when the concentration of atrazine (mixed with other pesticides) in water is highest, were more likely to have genital birth defects.

The author of the paper, Paul Winchester, a professor of pediatrics at the Indiana University School of Medicine, received a subpoena from Syngenta, which requested that he turn over every e-mail he had written about atrazine in the past decade. The company's media talking points described his study as 'so-called science' that didn't meet the 'guffaw test.' Winchester said, 'We don't have to argue that I haven't proved the point. Of course, I haven't proved the point! Epidemiologists don't try to prove points—they look for problems.'

A few months after Winchester's paper appeared, the Times published an investigation suggesting atrazine levels frequently surpass the maximum threshold allowed in drinking water. The article referred to recent studies in Environmental Health Perspectives and the Journal of Pediatric Surgery that found that mothers living close to water sources containing atrazine were more likely to have babies who were underweight or had a defect in which the intestines and other organs protrude from the body....

Hayes was confident that at the next E.P.A. hearing there would be enough evidence to ban atrazine, but in 2010 the agency found that the studies indicating risk to humans were too limited. Two years later, during another review, the E.P.A. determined that atrazine does not affect the sexual development of frogs. By that point, there were seventy-five published studies on the subject, but the E.P.A. exclude the majority of them from consideration, because they did not meet the requirements for quality that the agency had set in 2003. The conclusion was based largely on studies funded by Syngenta and led by Werner Kloss, a professor of endocrinology at Humboldt University in Berlin... One of the co-authors was Alan Hosmer, a Syngenta scientist whose job, according to a 2004 performance evaluation, included 'atrazine defense' and 'influencing EPA....'

NOTE: It was after this EPA hearing that the independent Boone Report was developed and released.

In another paper, in Policy Perspective, Jason Rohr, an ecologist at the University of South Florida, who served on an E.P.A. panel (with Michelle Boone, and subsequently contributing to the

Boone Report), *criticized the "lucrative 'science for hire' industry, where scientists are employed to dispute data." He wrote that a Syngenta-funded review of the atrazine literature had arguably misrepresented more than fifty studies and made a hundred and forty-four inaccurate or misleading statements, of which '96.5% appeared to be beneficial for Syngenta.' Rohr, who has conducted several experiments involving atrazine, said that, at conferences, 'I regularly get peppered with questions from Syngenta cronies trying to discount my research. They try to poke holes in the research rather than appreciate the adverse effects of the chemicals.' He said, 'I have colleagues whom I've tried to recruit, and they've told me that they're not willing to delve into this sort of research, because they don't want the headache of having to defend their credibility.'*

Deborah Cory-Slechta, a former member of the E.P.A's science advisory board, said that she, too, felt that Syngenta was trying to undermine her work. A professor at the University of Rochester Medical Center, Cory-Slechta studies how the herbicide paraquat may contribute to diseases of the nervous system. 'The folks from Syngenta used to follow me to my talks and tell me I wasn't using "human-relevant doses," she said. 'They would go up to my students and try to intimidate them. There was this sustained campaign to make it look like my science wasn't legitimate.'

The Growing Danger of Corporate Influence
Over Public Policies and Agrifood Systems

The dire issues of public health discussed herein are obviously not confined to the US and Canada, they are intensely global as noted in the report from Penang, Malaysia:[315]

Growing market concentration in multiple agricultural arenas, coupled with successive rounds of deregulation, have led to unprecedented levels of corporate influence over global and regional food and agricultural systems. As corporations based in Europe and North America have extended their operations into Latin America, Asia and Eastern Europe, their global influence has expanded, with

---

[315] Watts & Williamson, 204-205. Quoted and excerpted with permission.

adverse consequences for small and medium-scale farmers around the world. The result has been a dramatic reduction in competition and fair access to markets for small and medium-scale producers, labour, independent retailers and consumers.

The lack of adequate anti-trust and competition laws at national and international levels, and weak judicial systems that are unable to properly enforce existing laws have supported the unprecedented pace of corporate consolidation and adverse effects on family farming over the past two decades....

The world's largest corporations control over half (53%) of the world's commercial seed market; the top 10 control over three-quarters (76%) and one corporation (Monsanto) controls fully one quarter of the global market. This in turn has enabled them to exert significant political influence over public policy and research at national, regional and global levels, driving decisions and investment priorities consistently towards industrial models of agriculture that rely on the continual purchase of industry products such as chemical pesticides, fertilizers and patented seeds.

Agribusinesses spend billions of dollars lobbying public agencies and officials, in both national and international policy-making arenas, and have, in many instances, influenced policy decisions to their benefit. This influence undermines government resolve to launch country-wide transitions towards knowledge intensive agroecological farming practices that do not ensure continual sale of industry products. It also weakens government commitment to more strictly regulate commercial actors, remove perverse incentives that favour corporate profit over public interest, revise ownership laws and restore public access to and control over productive resources (e.g., seeds, land, water) that have been privatized.

Global trade has significant potential to support robust national and regional economies and drive a transition towards ecological agriculture. However, trade liberalization that has opened developing country markets to international competition too quickly or too extensively has undermined the rural sector and degraded the environment. As a result, developing countries have been left with diminished capacity for food production, making them more vulnerable to international food price and supply volatility, and reducing their food and livelihood security.

136

******

Bureaucratic Inertia

Very closely associated with collusion and co-optation is the simple malaise of bureaucratic inertia. A bureaucracy runs according to established routines within which those charged with the day-to-day responsibilities become systematically, if not systemically, accustomed to those rubrics of administration. Change does not come easily.

Change routinely encounters resistance, especially if personal and/or ideological interests are a stake. For example, as one mid-level E.P.A. official observed:

The same people who told us to ignore Safe Drinking Water Violations are still running the divisions. There's no accountability, and so nothing is going to change.[316]

Brown & Grossman note that their investigative research traces a "web of influence to a group of scientists working for the U.S. Department of Defense (DOD) in the 1970s and 1980s."[317] This group was the founders/inventors of PBPK (Physiologically Based Pharmacokinetics), a computer modeling simulation, originally utilized by the DOD. However, many of those DOD scientists discovered the PBPK "could be manipulated to minimize the appearance of chemical risk." And, that many of the inventors of PBPK "move between industry, government agencies, and industry-backed groups, often with little or no transparency."

The result? Chemicals which we are only recently learning are harmful, such as a variety of endocrine disruptors, continue to be "covered up" by EPA's adoption of the PBPK modeling enthusiastically adopted in-turn by chemical companies and the chemical industry-backed research agencies. Since PBPK relies solely on whatever data is fed into the computer (as do all computer simulations), "PBPK modeling can be deliberately manipulated to produce desired outcomes." In other words, the PBPK model can (and often is) tailor-made to provide exactly what Syngenta, Novartis Dow, Monsanto, or Dupont want to see.

---

[316] Duhigg, 3.
[317] Brown & Grossman.

University of Notre Dame biologist, Kristen Shrader-Frechette warns us that:

> *Models can offer a means of avoiding the conclusions derived from actual experiments.*

And, Leo Trasande, a NY University professor of medicine and health policy, cautions:

> *When you have biology telling you there are basic flaws in the model that's a compelling reason that It's time for a paradigm shift.*[318]

Collusion and co-optation, particularly as orchestrated by chemical companies, decisively influence regulatory agencies, and tramples individual, family, and community health and well-being. Sadness lies in the fact that we have come not only to accept the role of the fox at the door of the henhouse, we are condoning any collateral damage such as the so-called "guardianship" may render.

While we need to carefully examine and update PBPK, we must proceed with the awareness that there is a web of **undue** influence in which we must avoid being entangled. This web, unfortunately, has, since January 20, 2017, become intentional U.S. national policy, orchestrated from the West Wing of the White House where the evils of collusion and co-optation lead to unmitigated corruption; as well as massive harm to humanity.

---

[318] ibid. See also: Sharon Lerner, "EPA used Monsanto's Research to Give Roundup A Pass," The Intercept, November 3, 2015. https://theintercept.com/2015/11/03/epa-used-Monsantt-funded-research. Accessed December 9, 2015.

Chapter Nine:

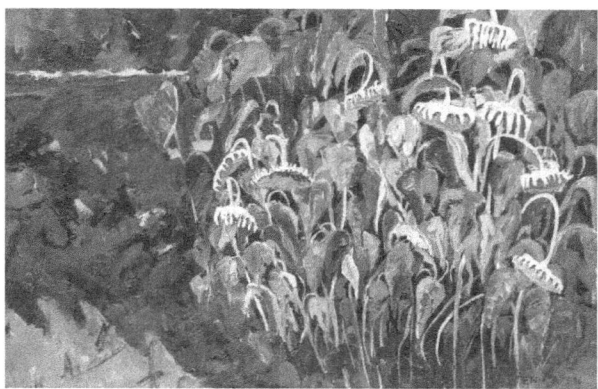

A Time to Mourn

Collateral Damage: Accepting the Unacceptable

> *We are dealing…with an absurdity that is not a quirk or an accident but is fundamental to our character as a people…the viciousness of a mentality that can look complacently upon disease as 'part of the cost' (*of being human).[319]
>
> (Wendell Berry)

As a nation, we seem to have resigned ourselves to cancer as a fact of life, that there is nothing we can do about it, and that pesticide use is as necessary as gasoline in the family car. If we are going to "get anywhere," we need gas in the car. If we are going to "get anywhere" with cropland farming, gardening, or lawn care, then we need to fill the land, the garden, or the lawn with pesticides.

As a nation we declared a "War on Pests" soon after World War II with little thought given to how creation is interlocked. Little-to-no critical thought was rendered regarding what we were unleashing. No attention was paid to the cost of life this war would exact on Nature itself and the delicate balance upon which life depends. No one in government (other than the lonely voice of Rachel Carson) seemed to care about the price in loss of life, due to this war, that would be billed directly to its people, in multiple and

---

[319] Wendel Berry, 18.

tragic ways.[320] Instead, a blind faith in science and technology welcomed, for example, DDT as "the War's greatest contribution to the future health of the world."[321]

Whenever the United States has considered going to war, there has usually been a public debate of some kind, an opportunity for some discussion about the need for such a war, its goals and objectives, its morality, its financial and human costs. Some such debate preceded engagement in the American Civil War, the Spanish American War, World War I and World War II, the Korean War, the Vietnam War, the War on Poverty, the War on Racism and Inequality, the Persian Gulf War, the US Response to the Attack Upon America in 2001 and, the 2003 American-Iraqi War.

Much of the debate preceding some US military engagements has swirled around the issue of keeping collateral, unintended, civilian casualties to a minimum. Some level of collateral damage is accepted as simply part of the cost of war. By one estimate anywhere from 214,000 to 265,000 Iraqi civilians were killed or later died because of US involvement in the Persian Gulf War.[322] The Iraq Body Count Organization estimates as of August 31, 2018, that 288,000 Iraqi civilians were killed as a result of the 2003 American invasion of their country and its on-going aftermath.[323] By another estimate approximately 1900 Panamanian citizens were killed and accepted as justifiable collateral damage when US forces successfully removed one man from power – General Manuel Noriega.[324]

Due to remoteness from the conflict thousands of miles across the ocean, and due to National Narcissism, we can accept those kinds of collateral damages. It's just the way war is. Regrettable, perhaps, but "unavoidable."

No discourse ever preceded the Chemical Warfare on Pests; perhaps because we believed and trusted our leaders' adage that we

---

[320] See Rachel Carson. (A PBS, An American Experience Production, 2017, 1:53 minutes.

[321] Brigadier General James Simmons, Saturday Evening Post, January 6, 1945 in Andrew Kimbrel, ed., The Fatal Harvest Reader: The Tragedy of Industrial Agriculture (Washington: Island Press, 2002), 92.

[322] Alan Geyer and Barbara G. Green, Lines in the Sand: Justice and the Gulf War (Louisville: Westminster/John Knox Press, 1992), 148-49.

[323] www.iraqbodycount.org. Accessed 7/12/2015.

[324] Noriega: God's Favorite (Showtime/Third Row Center Films, 2000).

would live better lives through science, especially the science of chemistry. As Sandra Steingraber plaintively puts it:

> *...as a member of the most poisoned generation to come of age, I am sorry that cooler heads did not prevail in the calm prosperity of peacetime, when careful consideration and a longer view on public health were once again permissible and necessary. I am sorry that no one asked, 'Is this the industrial path we want to continue along? ...Or that those who did ask such questions were not heard.*[325]

In other words, we drifted our way into acceptance of the Chemical Warfare on Pests similar to the manner of the chemical drifts that engulfed the croplands of America via aerial spraying and ground-based blowers as depicted the PBS documentary entitled Rachel Carson.[326]

While there is no denial that benefits from chemicals, can and do exist, one must take umbrage with their unbridled and detrimental use. No discernible debate was held regarding whether we should engage in chemical warfare upon so-called agricultural pests, to say nothing about any concern for what the collateral damages to human life and longevity might be. We wallowed in the euphoria that science would provide us with the good life. Perhaps no such debate occurred because as a nation we had already traveled beyond the limits of even caring.

For a nation that was the first (and, to date, the only) nation to use nuclear weapons, calculatingly accepting massive civilian casualties as part of the cost of eradicating the international pest known as the Japanese Empire, we may have gone beyond the limits of caring a whole lot about collateral damage. It does appear that such a stance is officially the way we do things as a country. In fact, all that is required is to consult the manual for exacting collateral damage.

---

[325] Steingraber # 1, 52, 115-116.
[326] Rachel Carson (A PBS "American Experience" Series Documentary), 2017; 113 minutes. CF 320.

Collateral Damage by the Book:
USAF Intelligence Targeting Guide, 1998

We seem to have developed official policy justifications, which inure us to the suffering brought on by our military actions. Witness the US Government's official guidebook on waging aerial and nuclear warfare, and the question of collateral human damage:

- *Collateral damage is unintentional damage or incidental damage… During Linebacker operations over North Vietnam, for example, some incidental damage occurred from bombs falling outside target areas. (Para. A7.1)*
- *Planning may also lead to maximizing collateral damage to enemy facilities near struck targets. (Para. A7.1.1)*
- *At a negligible risk distance, troops are fairly safe. Such a risk would be considered if nuclear weapons were to be used near friendly troops. Any greater risk would be accepted only when significant advantages could be gained. (Para.A7.2.1)*
- *At a moderate risk distance damage levels are tolerable, or at worst a minor nuisance. (Para. A7.2.2)*
- *When nuclear weapons are considered for employment against close-in targets, troop safety considerations may determine whether or not nuclear weapons will be used… As a rule, the commander will want a very high assurance (0.99 probability) that his troops will not be exposed to weapons effects higher than those considered acceptable. (Para. A7.4.1)*[327]

****

However, let it be known that the 1998 Intelligence Targeting Guide for assessing allowable nuclear collateral damage is hardly a new twist in American military strategy. The now-deceased Leonard Bird horrifically describes his own personal cost in being an unwilling and unwitting piece of nuclear collateral damage:

---

[327] "Attachment 7: Collateral Damage," <u>USAF Intelligence Targeting Guide</u> (Air Force Pamphlet 14-210 Intelligence, 1 February 1998), 179-183.
www.fas.org/irp/doddir/usaf/afpam14-210/part20.

In <u>Folding Paper Cranes: An Atomic Memoir</u>, [328] Bird graphically tells the story of being subjected to nuclear fallout while being marched into ditches at Yucca Flats as a Marine in the early 1950's. As a result of being so very close to ground zero more than once, Bird and his comrades were subjected to the radiation and radiated dust which they inhaled from the purposely detonated atomic bombs. He describes himself as a calculated piece of collateral damage[329] in that he and so many of his Marine companions at the time, have since contracted cancer, many of them dying at an early age. Bird's account is certainly of the same sad genre as Project Shad as noted in Chapter 2, in that they were military projects designed to use military personnel as human guinea pigs.

In October 2012, we learned that another military project chose to intentionally use the people of St. Louis, Missouri, U.S.A., in the same way, apparently with no regard for human collateral damage, In the 1960's and again in the 1970's, according to AP reporter Jim Salter,

...The Army used motorized blowers atop a low-income housing high-rise, at schools and from the backs of station wagons to send a potentially dangerous compound into the already-hazy air in predominantly black areas of St. Louis.[330]

Despite Salter's article which goes on to reveal anecdotal evidence of unusual incidents of cancer in the area where the tests were performed; and letters to Army Secretary John McHugh from Senators Claire McCaskill and Roy Blunt "demanding answers," as of this writing, the proverbial jury is still out. The Army did an investigation and reported November 2012 that the chemicals used posed no risk to the people of St. Louis. However, the sociologist who conducted the original research, Lisa Martino-Taylor, remains un-reassured. She claims that she had seen way too much "secrecy

---

[328]

[329] Ibid, 32-55.

[330] Jim Salter, "Report: Army tested chemical weapons on St. Louis in 1950's," October 4, 2012, Knox News.
www.knoxnews.com/news/2012/oct/04/repoer/report-army-tested-chemical-weapons.

and deception," to accept without reservations the Army's denial of any public health issue due to the 1950's chemical tests.[331]

It is not the intent here to engage in an in-depth analysis of US military strategies. This writer only wishes to demonstrate the parallel between US policy on doing what it takes to eradicate the human enemy in war and eradication of pests in the croplands of America, tossing collateral damage to the nuclear and chemical winds.

As paragraph A7.1 of the USAF Intelligence Targeting Guide points out, collateral damage, while it may be "unintentional," is to be seen as simply "incidental." Wiping out an entire village by a "misguided" "Smart Bomb," while "unintentional" is simply an "incidental" event, an event of little consequence, "a minor nuisance." While the introduction of DDT and the various triazines into the environment, onto the land, into the water table, and mixed into the air we breathe, was not intended to cause cancer, Government and Corporate America seem to hold the attitude that the damage done to the Donna Jos is simply incidental, of little consequence in the long view. Indeed, "a minor nuisance."

If we, as a nation, are prepared to launch another nuclear war, as noted in Paragraph A7.4.1, even if it means putting our own troops at risk at some unidentified level of acceptance; if, as James Douglass claims in his book, JFK and the Unspeakable,[332] Kennedy's Joint Chiefs of Staffs (unknown to the President) planned a nuclear first strike attack on Cuba and Russia with no regard given to the innocent citizens who would suffer much more than the Japanese in 1945, then what is the big deal about putting a few people at risk with carcinogenic-laden pesticides in rural America?

The deal is this: as a nation we are at risk of losing our soul. A soulless nation that, by definition, has become "devoid of sensitivity or the capacity of deep feeling."[333] When the US Military

---

[331] Veronica Lacapra, "Army: Cold War Chemical Weapons Testing Posed No Risk to St. Louisans," St. Louis Public Radio, November 2, 2012. http://news.stlpublicradio.org/post/army-cold-war-chemical-weapons-testing-posed-no-risk-st-louisans#stream/0. Accessed September 3, 2018.

[332] James W. Douglass, JFK and the UNSPEAKABLE: Why He Died & Why It Matters (Maryknoll, NY: Orbis Books, 2008), 235.

[333] The American Heritage Dictionary.

Command opted for a deforestation policy in Vietnam – a policy driven by the desire to exterminate the enemy at all costs, we exposed the enemy to napalm and Agent Orange; AND countless numbers of Vietnamese families suffered.[334] So, too, we incurred countless numbers of collateral damage to the lives of our own troops. Duane was one of them:

Lieutenant Farmer Duane's Story

Duane (1951-2000), a 49-year-old Vietnam War veteran dying of massive cancer invasion most likely caused by Agent Orange, issued the opinion one day that "my name should be on the Vietnam Wall in DC. I'm just a late casualty, that's all."

Far be it for this author to question Duane's assessment that his name should be on the Vietnam Memorial Wall. Far be it for me to question Duane's sense that he was "just a piece of collateral damage" from the debris of the Vietnam War. Unfortunately, Duane's contribution to the Vietnam War casualty list, even as a cipher, may never be entered in any War Almanac.

Unfortunately, Duane may never have stood a chance of overcoming the effects of Agent Orange, even by returning home to the family farm in Iowa. Duane's experience of having been raised on a farm in the Nishna "valley was very similar to Donna Jo and the other women featured in this book. Is it possible that Duane had already developed Multiple Chemical Sensitivity even before enlisting in the US Army? Is it possible that Duane's exposure to DDT, 2-4D, and the triazine pesticides predisposed him to an extreme reaction to Agent Orange in either or both of his two tours in Vietnam? It is conceivable that Duane was collateral damage looking for a place to happen as he left the farm for Vietnam and as he left Vietnam to return to the farm.

Perhaps in the long and aggregate view, Duane's death is but an "incidental" one. Even if he were to be counted as a Vietnam War

---

[334] "Three Vietnamese victims of Agent Orange have begun legal action against...more than 20 American companies...including Dow Chemical Co. and Monsanto Co." (Legal Action by Vietnamese Agent Orange Victims was Inevitable," World AFP, February 3, 2003. www.panna.org.

casualty, the War Room strategists would certainly count Duane's death as an "incidental" loss. But, again, do we really care?

When the USS was ruthlessly attacked by the Israeli Air force and Navy on June 8, 1967,[335] President Lyndon Johnson directed his commander of the Sixth Fleet in the Mediterranean that he "didn't care if the ship sunk, he would not embarrass his allies."[336] The USS Liberty was considered expendable collateral damage, a reasonable price to pay to save "embarrassing our allies"—who were only trying to cover-up their atrocity at El Arish, Egypt, where civilians and POWs were systematically slaughtered. But was it a "reasonable price" to pay for the 34 families whose loved ones died and the 171 families whose loved ones were wounded on that ship?[337]

Is Duane's death a reasonable price to be paid by his family? Maybe, just maybe, Duane's death, to the extent it may have been due to Agent Orange, could be seen as a reasonable cost IF Agent Orange had won the war for the US. Some would argue that the end justifies the means. However, Agent Orange failed miserably in its objectiv4 and succeeded only in killing countless non-combatants and desecrating the land.

The unbridled use of agrichemicals in the interest of maximizing cropland production took, as expendable collateral damage, the lives of Donna Jo, Sandra, JoAn, Shelley, Helen and Ben, and Duane. But do we care? Massive evidence suggests we do not.

The National Center for Policy Analysis (NCPA) Report notes that the "median toxic control program costs 146 times more per life saved than the median medical intervention."[338] The implied conclusion is that we should give it up, accept the collateral damage, and move on. It is cheaper to treat cancer than to prevent it from proliferating.

The coup de grace for this argument is the estimated $140 billion per year cost incurred by government to administer

---

[335] James Bamford, <u>Body of Secrets: Anatomy of the Ultra-Secret National Security Agency from the Cold War Through the Dawn of a New Century</u> (NY: Doubleday, 2001), 185-239.
[336] Ibid, 226.
[337] Ibid, 201.
[338] NCPA, Executive Summary #4

environmental regulations.[339] There is, of course, no consideration given to the possibility that if pesticides were simply made illegal, we could make a $140 billion per year savings; and, in doing so save millions of lives – as well as save millions more from the pain of losing loved ones to what could have been preventable death. Instead, NCPA argues that the only way to go is to "set priorities based on cost-effectiveness in order to save the most lives,"[340] and the priorities suggested by NCPA would include redirecting attention to the carcinogens produced by Mother Nature; and forget about any corporate-made cancer-causing products.

The case of Dr. Omar Shafey indicates that collateral damage in the pesticide wars is not just tolerated; it is a matter of public policy. However, it is a silent, nefarious, and democratically indefensible policy. The case of Dr. Shafey illustrates so very clearly how it is that even regulatory agencies charged with protecting public health have been corrupted. Politics, cost-benefit analysis and profit motives claim first priorities over people, communities and families. The lives, hopes and dreams of the Donna Jo's, Sandra's, and Susans are placed on the balance sheet and are found unimportant or insignificant. The loss of those lives, hope, and dreams are considered incidental losses, expendable, disposable – all in the interest of not wanting to embarrass such allies as *Allied Chemical Incorporated.*

Is it not time to "declare a 'cease fire' and transform modern food production from the war against the land to a marriage of ecology and agriculture?"[341]

---

[339] Ibid.
[340] NCPA Report, Misconception # 10.
[341] Kimbrel, 92, 103.

Chapter Ten:

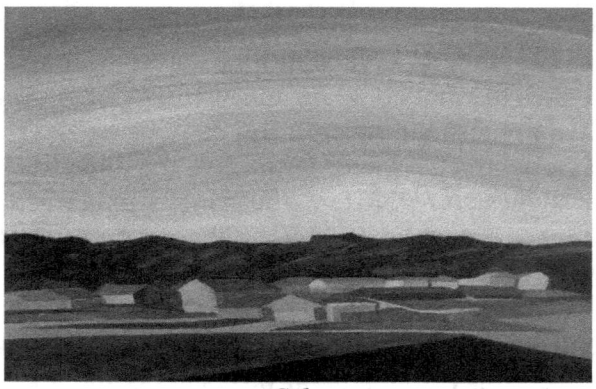

Calm

The Precautionary Principle: Do No Harm
(Or: An Ounce of Pesticides is Worth a Pound of Precaution)

Scientific uncertainty is no excuse for inaction…
We cannot wait for 'proof.'
(Siddhartha Mukherjee)[342]

At a 1987 meeting concerning the environmental and ecological damage being done to the North Sea, European representatives, holding portfolios for their governments, adopted the Precautionary Principle as one of their major modes of moving forward.[343] This principle gives precedence and preference to public safety, and public health, as well as preservation of the environment and caution; or, as Sandra Steingraber notes:

---

[342] Siddhartha Mukherjee, The Emperor of All Maladies: A Biography of Cancer(NY: Scribner, 2010), 424,

[343] K. Geiser, "The Greening of Industry: Making the Transition to a Sustainable Economy," Technology Review, August-September 1991, 65-72; T. O'Riordan and J. Cameron (eds.), Interpreting the Precautionary Principle (London: Earthscan, 1994).

The Precautionary Principle…dictates that indication of harm, rather than proof of harm, should be the trigger for action – especially if delay may cause irreparable damage.[344]

Pope Francis addresses this principle by drawing attention to the Rio declaration of 1992 which states:

Where there are threats of serious or irreversible damage, lack of full scientific, certainty shall not be used as a pretext for postponing cost-effective measures which prevent environmental degradation. This precautionary principle makes it possible to protect those who are most vulnerable and whose ability to defend their interests and to assemble incontrovertible evidence is limited. If objective information suggests that serious and irreversible damage may result, a project should be halted or modified, even in the absence of indisputable proof. Here the burden of proof is effectively reversed, since in such cases objective and conclusive demonstrations will have to be brought forward to demonstrate that the proposed activity will not cause serious harm to the environment or to those who inhabit it.[345]

If the Precautionary Principle had guided the US Government in granting pesticide licenses from the beginning, the chemical companies would have been required to scientifically prove the public safety of their products and withstand the scrutiny of government-sponsored private research aimed at verifying the safety of those same chemicals. Instead, the American approach seems to be to grant a license first and worry about a public health problem later, if at all. The operative principle might be called the Principle of Hoping-for-the-Best, with its own corollary: Keep-Your-Fingers-Crossed!

Quite in contrast to American Farm Bureau Federation evaluations of pesticides on public health is the testimony and tragic personal story of Dr. Nicole Bruinsma, a Quebec family physician who herself had been diagnosed with breast cancer. Dr. Bruinsma

---

[344] Steingraber # 1, 270; # 2. 281-82.
[345] Pope Francis, 186; citing the Rio Declaration on the Environment and Development (14 June 1992, Principle 15. 137. www.iisd.org/rio+5/agenda/declaration.htm. Accessed July 18, 2015.

appeared before the Canadian House of Commons Committee on the Environment claiming that "there is enough evidence linking pesticides to breast cancer to justify adopting a precautionary approach for their use. 'How much evidence is enough?'" she asked.[346]

The prevailing "answer" to Dr. Bruinsma's rather rhetorical question is well-stated by Dr. Sandra Steingraber, also a victim of cancer, who claims:

I am more concerned that the uncertainty over details is being used to call into doubt the fact that profound connections do exist between human health and the environment. I am more concerned that uncertainty is too often parlayed into an excuse to do nothing until more research can be conducted.[347]

Furthermore, it is to be noted that Steingraber goes on to conclude:

'We need more study' is the grandfather of all arguments for taking no action... "[348]

*****

The Case of Dr. Nicole Bruinsma (1960-2002)

Nicole Bruinsma, MD, happily married, mother of three young girls, a health & fitness "nut," was diagnosed with breast cancer in 1997 at the age of 37. With four good reasons (her daughters and husband), she was determined to beat the cancer. Almost immediately, she had one breast removed, followed by radiation treatment, and then chemotherapy. Following the old rule of "it's better to be safe than sorry," she had the remaining breast removed, as a precautionary attempt to ward off the cancer.

Since there was no history of cancer in her birth family, Bruinsma set out to find the cause for the battle in which she found

---

[346] "Breast Cancer and Pesticide Link," Beyond Pesticides Daily News Archive, April 8, 2002. www.beyondpesticides.org/NEWS/dailynewsarchive/040802.html.
[347] Steingraber # 1, 72-73, # 2, 71.
[348] Steingraber # 1, 73; Citing P.F. Infante and G.K. Pohl, "Living in a Chemical World: Actions and Reactions to Industrial Carcinogens," Teratogenesis, Carcinogenesis and Mutagenesis8 (1998): 225-49.

herself engaged. That same year (1997), she attended the First World Conference on Breast Cancer held at Queen's University in Kingston, Ontario. At the conference, she viewed the documentary film Exposure,[349] that strongly suggested pesticides could cause cancer through endocrine disruption and estrogen dysfunction. The film appears to have been a "game-changer" for Dr. Bruinsma.[350] From that moment to the end of her life, she devoted herself to the elimination of pesticides.

While the cancer did go into remission, by 2000 it had returned with a vengeance. However, despite the metastasizing cancer, Nicole was doubly determined to beat the monster. She had her ovaries removed and endured more chemotherapy. She was offered the possibility of using the chemical Taxotere. Since it was manufactured by the Aventis Corporation, Bruinsma was thrown into an ethical dilemma: she would be using and paying for a drug produced by a company that produces pesticides. It would be a cruel irony, that the very company, perhaps, that manufactured the causal agent of her cancer would provide the antidote, if not the cure. She initially refused, but in a "Last Hurrah" effort, she finally agreed to the Taxotere treatment. Miraculously, it worked, for a short while. Nicole died on February 27, 2002, five agonizing years after her initial diagnosis.

Due, in large part, to Nicole's activism against pesticides, the influence of the Canadian Association of Physicians for the Environment (which she helped found), and the publicity surrounding her death, the large Canadian retail chain, Loblaw Companies, announced in 2002 it would no longer sell chemical pesticides in any of its 440 garden centers. To date the following provinces have either banned or severely restricted the use of pesticides:

- Alberta
- British Columbia
- New Brunswick

---

[349] Rooney Productions, "Who was Nicole Bruinsma? Why is this story so Important?" http://www.precautionaryprinciplefilm.com/project-in-depth.html Cited hereafter as "Who was Nicole Bruinsma?"

[350] Exposure: Environmental Links to Breast Cancer. Available through Women's Healthy Environments Network (WHEN). www.womenshealthyenvironments.ca/films.

- Newfoundland & Labrador
- Nova Scotia
- Ontario
- Quebec[351]

Two years later (2008), Home Depot and Walmart announced they, too, were eliminating pesticide from their inventories.[352]

Of course, the chemical companies have not rolled over in defeat. Dow Chemical Company took the lead in challenging the bans in accord with DOW's understanding of NAFTA[353] (the North American Fair Trade Agreement). On May 25, 2011, a non-monetary settlement was reached between Dow chemical and the Province of Quebec. Both Dow and supporters of the ban claim victory. Supporters believe the settlement establishes the right of provinces and municipalities to codify their own pesticide ordinances. Dow claims Quebec has agreed, "a popular weed killer can be used properly without health risks."[354] However, the settlement allows Quebec to retain Dow's pesticide on the Province's banned list.

*****

Medical Ethics: A Guide to Safe and Responsible Use of Pesticides

One would presume, a government concerned about its nation's health and safety would want to be reasonably sure a given toxic chemical is in fact safe before allowing it onto the market place and into the environment and food supply. A government conscientiously concerned about the common good and general welfare of its people would be guided by the medical ethic on Non-Malfeasance, or do no harm. This government would be alert to avoiding harm; and, this

---

[351] Coalition for Alternatives to Pesticides-NL.
http://pesticidealternativesnl.wordpress.com/rest-of-canada
[352] "Who was Nicole Bruinsma?"
[353] See Naomi Klein, This Changes Everything: Capitalism vs. The Climate (NY: Simon & Schuster, 2014, 83-85, especially, for a discussion of NAFTA as a tragic event for the health and welfare of the world.
[354] "NAFTA pesticide ban challenge settled without money," CBC News-Montreal (May 30, 2011) www.cbc.ca/ndews/canada/montreal/vafta-pesticide-ban-challenge-settled-without-money-1.1005002.

government would pursue another ethic of medical practice – always pursuing the Less Invasive Means of solving a problem.

It is not the intent here to glorify the medical community as "holier than thou." Clearly, individual physicians have violated both the ethics of Non-Malfeasance and Less Invasive Means. In doing so those same doctors violated the Precautionary Principe as well. There will be no argument here defending physicians who may well have intentionally infracted all three codes of conduct for less than morally acceptable reasons.

Certainly, physicians have made medical intervention decisions that were:

- A rush to judgment – such as opting immediately for prostate surgery rather than pursuing other avenues (such as "watching it"), therefore violating the Precautionary Principle.
- Most Invasive – such as the above example, therefore violating the ethic of Less Invasive Means.
- More harmful to the patient than no treatment at all – such as holding out false hope to a clearly terminal patient and pursuing aggressive chemo therapy up to the point of death, thereby violating the ethic Non-Malfeasance.
- Imposed upon the patient without their consent or knowledge – such as ordering or performing CPR on a patient having a cardiac arrest, despite knowing that the patient has an Advanced Directive ordering that there be no resuscitation or intubation – thereby violating yet another ethic: the ethic of Patient Autonomy.[355]

For a rather graphic narrative describing medical practices that violated every modern notion of ethical, responsible, and compassionate care for cancer patients, see especially Mukherjee's chapter entitled, "A Radical Idea."[356] All done in accordance with the prevailing ethic: "Preserve Life at All Costs."

The ethic of Patient Autonomy maintains that the patient, or those designated to make decisions for the patient, is informed about

---

[355] See the film Witt, starring Emma Thompson, based on Margaret Edison's 1997 Pulitzer prize winning play (HBO Studios, DVD, 2004.
[356] Mukherjee, 60-72; plus, the first two pages of photos.

the nature and consequences of medical intervention, and that the patient (or patient's surrogate) renders his/her consent.

Instead of being guided by these principles and ethics, our government and the vested interests within our governing structure are guided by the Principle of Profit. The latter comes with its own corollary: that which is profitable, is therefore safe and good. The Precautionary Principle's corollary is: that which is safe, is therefore good and may (or may not) be profitable.

The Precautionary Principle throws the burden of proof on those who would introduce a new chemical into the environment. The producer would be required to prove safety. Currently it is up to the public to prove there is a breach of public health and safety. The parallel in Anytown, USA, would be to require those involved in an accident to prove "Joe Candidate's huge sign inches from the curb at the intersection of First & Main did in fact cause the accident. Meanwhile, as court litigation proceeds at a typical snail's pace the signage stays in place continuing to be a public hazard – and the "accidents" pile up at the intersection of Politics and Public Safety.

Unfortunately, we have a long and inglorious history of violating, ignoring and discounting the Precautionary Principle in the area of public health. Surgeon General Luther Terry announced on January 12, 1964 that his efforts to deal with the hazards of cigarette smoke for public health would be guided by the assumption that the scientific studies point to cause and effect relationships, and that he would not hold off regulating the cigarette industry until such time that absolutely no uncertainty exists.[357] It was not until a courageous whistleblower (scientist, Jeffrey Wigand) from inside the cigarette giant Brown & Williamson Cigarette Company spoke out 34 years later, that serious action was taken against an industry that was not just complicit in a somewhat less-than innocent act, but an industry that was guilty of wreaking intentional harm on the consumers of its products.[358]

As Dr. Janette Sherman notes:

We knew about the toxicity of asbestos in 1898, about benzene's hazards in 1862, the predicted carcinogenicity of DES in 1938, and the certainty of DDT's harm in 1952. But we allowed the

---

[357] Sherman # 1, 207
[358] The Insider (1999). See also Mukherjee, 238-455.

'experts' to do 'one more study,' and allowed the interests of business to come before those of the public.[359]

There are those, of course, who oppose the Precautionary Principle from a variety of practical, political, and philosophical perspectives. The political scientist, Dr. Aaron Wildavsky, for example, in discussing worst-case risk assessment, contends:

We should be guided by the probability and extent of harm, not by its mere possibility… The past necessity of proving harm has been replaced by a reversal of causality: now the individuals and businesses must prove that they will do no harm. My objection to this… is profound: our liberties are curbed and our health is harmed.[360]

Along the same line of argument, we find Chris (C.F.) Wilkinson saying:

It is important to consider obsession with identifying, regulating, and generally worrying about what often appear to be trivial carcinogenic risks associated with many synthetic chemicals against the truly overwhelming background of natural carcinogens.[361]

The Wildavsky and Wilkinson arguments fit snugly into the pocket of those who would continue manufacturing, distributing, and applying toxic substances to the environment with little to no regard for their impact upon human health, leaving the gates of collusion, complicity and corruption wide open.

Without the Precautionary Principle in place, cooptation leads almost naturally to collusion between government and business, or any ingrained and politically influential interest. One potential sign of the collusion is the fact that while old untested pesticides were required to be scientifically assessed by 1976, the

---

[359] Sherman, 209.
[360] A.B. Wildavsky, But is it True? A Citizen's Guide to Environmental Health and Safety (Cambridge: Harvard University Press, 1995).
[361] Chris Wilkinson, "Being More Realistic About Chemical Carcinogenesis," 3.

deadline was delayed for at least a quarter century![362] In the meantime, all of the untested chemicals remain on the market – and the "accidents" pile up at the intersection of Safety and Profit.

Even with the Precautionary Principle in place, care needs to be taken to assure that completely neutral parties perform testing. A careful screening process must replace the common practice of government agencies relying on, for example, Syngenta's scientific reports, or going to universities heavily funded by various chemical companies. Current practice violates the conflict of interest ethic. Relying upon the chemical industry to inform us od the safety of its own products is like having a funeral director on a medical ethics committee deciding whether or not more aggressive treatment is justified for a particular patient. The current practice is the same as having end-of-life issues totally in the hands of the funeral industry – and all of the evidence being buried with the deceased.

Along with the Precautionary Principle comes the need to invoke stricter standards of safety. Public Safety Disclosures must abandon the category labeled: **There is Lack of Evidence of Harm.** Too easily consumers translate this as meaning: **This Chemical is Safe; This Chemical has been Certified as Harmless.**

A stricter standard would call government and the chemical industry to side with the ethic of Non-Malfeasance assuring that no harm would come to the user or innocent bystanders. A stricter standard would also lead to a fuller respect for the ethic of Patient, or in this case, Citizen Autonomy. The potential user of the chemical would be informed of known potential hazards. However, for the sake of the common good there needs to be one more very important principle invoked based on the ethic of Less Invasive Means – The Principle of the Least Toxic Alternative.[363]

---

[362] L. Ember, "Pollution Prevention: Study Says Chemical Industry Lags," Chemical and Engineering News, 20 March 1995, 6. Sherman notes that EPA does NOT regulate or directly study chemical toxicity, it merely registers products based on evidence presented by the chemical industry – and all the evidence is classified as "business confidentiality" or "unpublished." (204)
[363] Steingraber # 1, 271.

The Principle of the Least Toxic Alternative

This principle dictates a measure of government regulation that will immediately strike the conservative-capitalist as anathema. It would require that someone other than the individual homeowner, family farmer, or agribusiness do the evaluative assessment regarding the least toxic approach to solving a problem. Licensed pesticide evaluators would become common fixtures, and no pesticides could be purchased or applied anywhere, whether on lawns or cropland without documented, certified, licensed approval by a Licensed Pesticide-Use Evaluator.

At risk of sounding like a Yogi Berra Zen philosopher, unless we change the way we do things, the way we do things will not change. The way we are currently using chemical pesticides on food and field crops is killing us. Until we adopt the Precautionary Principe, the Principle of Least Toxic Alternatives and the medical ethics of Non-Malfeasance, Citizen/Patient Autonomy, and Least Invasive Means, we as a nation stand guilty of crimes against humanity. The practice of purchasing and applying the most toxic alternative available, while creating potential for the most invasive threat to human health and impacting people who have had no knowledge of the implications for their own, their family's or their community's health constitutes what amounts to chemical warfare on our own people.

As Sandra Steingraber prophetically pleads:

The principle of the least toxic alternative looks toward the day when the availability of safer choices makes the deliberate and routine release of chemical carcinogens into the environment as unthinkable as the practice of slavery.[364]

Certainly, there are features of pesticide use that are similar to slavery:

- We have become slaves ourselves as we become enslaved to pesticide use, enslaved in the pursuit of the next most effective (that is, the most toxic/"effective") pesticide.

---

[364] Ibid, # 2, 283.

- Our neighbors, without their consent or knowledge become enslaved, oppressed by our choices.
- The health of our own families and that of our neighbors is held in bondage to our choices.

The truly sad component to this tragic waste of the earth and human health is that it is so avoidable. The chemical warfare we are waging on one another, this crime against humanity that we condone, this victimization in which we are all complicit harkens back to an Aristotelian wisdom that we seem never to learn:

The greatest crimes are committed not for the sake of necessities, but for the sake of the superfluities.[365]

The bottom line must be the protection of human health. At least 50 municipalities in Canada banned or severely restricted pesticide use on public and private properties. In 2001 the Canadian Supreme Court ruled that these municipal ordinances are lawful. Proof of cause and effect, according to this ruling, is NOT required. All that is needed to justify such bans or restrictions is, according to the court, public perception that a problem exists:

If the public perceives that they are at risk from a certain chemical, they can act to protect themselves.[366]

In modern American political and military parlance, the Canadian Supreme Court condones "Pre-emptive Warfare" on pesticides. The court has come down on the side of "playing it safe" when it comes to the health and welfare of the Canadian people. The judges have recognized that the available date is less than definitive, but their opinion is entirely in line with the call by the authors of Our Stolen Future:

---

[365] Ernest Barker, ed & trans, The Politics of Aristotle (Oxford University Press, 1962), 66, VII. II.
[366] Beyond Pesticides, "Community Group Fights for Lawn Pesticide Ban," January 9, 2004.

Given the nature of the contamination, it is important to recognize at the outset that those responsible for safeguarding human health will have to act on information that is less than perfect… As we wrestle with the question of how much chemical contaminants are contributing to the trends…we see in breast cancer, prostate disease, infertility, and learning disabilities – it is important to keep one thing in mind. Scientists keep finding significant, often permanent effects at surprisingly low doses. The danger we face is not simply death and disease. By disrupting hormones and development, these synthetic chemicals may be changing who we become, they may be altering our destinies.[367]

The Canadian Court has joined the Superior Administrative Court of Cundinamaca, Columbia, which ruled on June 25, 2003 that "the significant and potentially irreparable risk posed by…spraying is reason enough to suspend the fumigation program" of herbicide aerial spraying to destroy coca and poppy crops."[368]

If the above principles, with an accompanying strict standard of safety enforcement, had been in place in 1940, the chances are Donna Jo, Sandra, Susan, JoAn, Shelley, and Duane, would all be alive today. Now, however, 70 years later, light has come to bear on the issues related here from a critical source at the top, so to speak, as noted by NY Times columnist Nicholas Kristof who claims: "The President's Cancer Panel is the Mount Everest of the medical mainstream" and that overall the 2010 Report is "astonishing."[369]

Perhaps the main reason Kristof finds the report "astonishing" is that its number one "Policy and Program Recommendation" calls for the invocation of the Precautionary Principle. In doing so, the PCP identifies a long list of "Responsible Agencies, Stakeholders, and Other Entities" for carrying out this recommendation. Those listed Range from the President and Congress on down to state governments and industry.[370]

---

[367] Our Stolen Future, 197.
[368] "Columbia Court Orders Suspension of Coca Spraying," Earthjustice, June 26, 2003. www.earthjustice.org/news/print.html?ID=620.
[369] Nicholas Kristof, ""New Alarm Bells About Chemicals and Cancer," New York Times, May 6, 2010.
[370] PCP 2010, xi.

Dr. Meriel Watts and the Pesticide Action Network go one step further with a more global view of the urgency for prevention of the calamity of cancer:

It is imperative that we apply the precautionary principle...and dramatically reduce women's exposure to pesticides that may be contributing to the escalating global epidemic of breast cancer.[371]

Complicity:
We Have Seen the Enemy and the Enemy is Us

Going back to first instances, we may see that the Donna Jos troubles began years before being diagnosed with cancer. They had been repeatedly exposed to pesticides in the air they breathed, the water they drank, and the food they ate, without their knowledge or consent. It was the choices others made that gave these women no choice whatever but to follow the path of pain and a shortened life – choices made by others for the most toxic alternative.

Many people and institutions (public and private) were complicit in the death of these women, and millions like them. To be complicit in an act generally takes one of the following forms:

- Willful and knowledgeable intent: But no one willfully and with intentional knowledge caused Donna Jo or Sandra's death.
- Willful and knowledgeable negligence: A doctor who may have intentionally kept important information away from Susan or JoAn may be so charged here.

However, chemical companies that persist in marketing carcinogenic products despite mounting scientific evidence that says there is a public health hazard are to be charged with the highest indictment for the death of millions of other people. A government that turns its head allowing these death-dealing products to continue their destructive path invites the highest distrust of its people. Both government and chemical corporations may one day even be found guilty of the highest form of crime: being accessories in the death of

---

[371] Watts, 16.g

millions of people across the country and world—CRIMES AGAINST HUMANITY

If only the Precautionary Principle and the other principles/ethics cited here had been deployed, Susan and millions of others would have at least had the opportunity to live longer and with much less painful lives. But, we cannot go back and re-set the clock. We cannot return to the past and take the road not travelled. We can, however, go back to the future.

Back to the Future

By going "back to the future" we do not mean a replication of the fantasy movie by the same name, Nor, does it imply finding some miraculous vehicle which, if we can just its speed up to a certain mark we will, as the fictional Dr. Emmett L. Brown states, "see some serious shit!"[372] Rather, we do have the means of re-examining the past and re-assessing the present. As we do so, we must be prepared for the depressing discovery that our life-style and actions indict us in our own complicity in the chemical warfare unleashed against ourselves.

If such an examination of national conscience is going to have any redeeming value at all, it cannot linger in the past or the present; it must look to the future. Such examination of social conscience must be aimed at a more sustainable future. A sustainable future requires that we stop the killing: the killing of the land; the killing of the environment; and the killing of one another. We must stop killing ourselves.

As a society we are unintentional accessories to homicide, and suicidal with o accompanying suicidal ideation.[373] The same is true at the individual as well as the corporate level – up to a point.

---

[372] Dr. Emmett L. Brown, The eccentric scientist in the film Back to the Future (1985).

[373] By "suicidal ideation" we mean the expression verbally or non-verbally of the wish, the evidence of a plan, and perhaps possessing the means to end one's life. Clearly, no one who persists in the use of carcinogenic pesticides even indirectly indicates a suicidal ideation. Yet, practically speaking, such continued use, given what we know about the effects on human health, comes down to a form of suicidal intent.

The demarcation line that separates conscious intent from the unintentional is the all-important element known as knowledge.

The Idaho potato grower who told Michael Pollan that he would never put potatoes from his cash crop on his own family table because of the pesticides he uses[374] would be open to a charge of being a willful and intentional accessory to homicide. If he were to hold the same opinion regarding the harmful effects of those pesticides and placed his cash crop potatoes on his family's table, a case could be made that perhaps he was non-verbally expressing suicidal ideation; at the very least he could be charged with willful neglect of his family's health and welfare.

The farmer who continues using carcinogenic chemicals despite his or her knowledge of the deleterious effect on public health, and the corporations that continue marketing these substances despite warnings issued by scientific research, are both subject to the charge of placing the public in grave danger. The corporation that intentionally manipulates research findings in order to put their products in unjustifiable good lights is the corporation that has crossed the line from unintentionality into that of a public crime, if not a crime against humanity. The scientist who appears to have sold his/her soul, bending the truth to protect a corporation's product and profit has, well, sold his/her soul.

As Wendell Berry notes, "That no sane creature befouls its own nest is accepted as generally true."[375] True, perhaps, for all creatures except for humankind! The Library of Congress estimates that 4,400,000,000 pounds of DDT were laid upon the human nest just in the United States from 1940 to 1993.[376] As noted previously the sale and use of atrazine/simazine as produced by Geigy Chemical Corporation increased over 4000% between 1959 and 1960.[377]

Thomas Berry sums it up by saying, when the "earth community" is treated "in an abusive way a vengeance awaits the human, for when the other living species are violated so extensively, the human itself is imperiled."[378] This writer does not intend to delve

---

[374] CF 9, Chapter 5.

[375] Wendell Berry, 51.

[376] Regenstein, 338.

[377] Fagan, 18.

[378] Thomas Berry, The Dream of the Earth (San Francisco: Sierra Club Books, 1988), 2.

into how our use of pesticides has created horrendous damage to the ecology, to bird, fish, and animal and plant life. The intent here is to focus on the damage we are doing to ourselves. Yet, as Thomas Berry suggests, the damage we do to the land, the environment, and to the ecology, we do unto ourselves. He also observes that:

If evil persons with destructive intentions did the assault on the earth, it would be understandable. The tragedy is that our economy is being run by persons with good intentions under the illusion that they are bringing only great benefits to the world and even fulfilling a sacred task on the part of the human community.[379]

While it is true that business, corporations, banks, Wall Street, Madison Avenue, and government "run" the economy, it is also "run" by us, the consumer. Whether we are the farmer seeking the most effective method of controlling pests toward the end of maximizing crop production, or the gardener seeking the same end for one's garden, or the homeowner seeking the same end for a rich green lawn, our choices lay a heavy hand on running the economy. As Pogo once said, "We have seen the enemy and the enemy is us!"

But it is most uncommon for us to see ourselves as the enemy. The enemy is always "out there," beyond our selves. In the case addressed here, the enemy is most commonly identified as the pests. What we are really saying is that the enemy is nature itself.

Unfortunately, we have resigned ourselves to fighting that supposed enemy with whatever means available. Worse yet, we have accepted that there will be "collateral damage." We never entertain the idea, however, that the collateral damage will be done unto our families, our neighbors, our communities, our nation, our world or ourselves. At best, we may rationalize the casualties as victims of "friendly fire."

---

[379] Ibid, 77.

Chapter Eleven

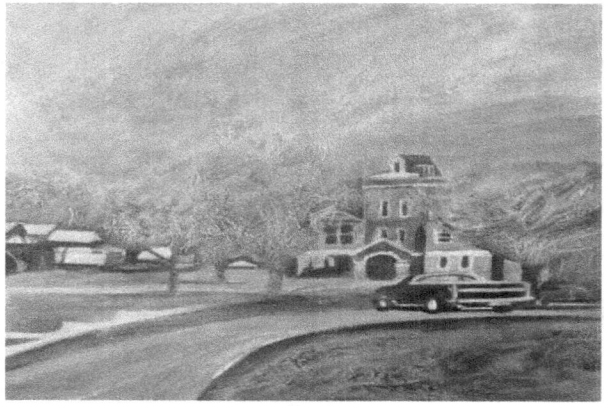

Sleet

Preoccupation with Downstream Symptoms versus Upstream Precipitators

So often, indeed most of the time, we become so preoccupied with the symptoms downstream in our lives that we neglect to look upstream for the causes. Frequent experiences of "heartburn," for example, cause us to run to the cupboard for Pepto-Bismol, Tums, or a quick fix with baking soda. Even a physician's diagnosis of acid reflux often does not produce a hard look at the upstream precipitator, i.e., eating too much of the wrong kinds of food at the wrong time of the day.

The same is true for cancer. We simply accept the cancer casualties as normal without looking for upstream causes. Worse yet, we sometimes identify other downstream flotsam as causal factors, when they are in fact incidental tributaries to the content of the larger stream.

Cancer & Heredity: Up the Creek Without a Paddle

Much has been done in the area of hereditary predilection toward cancer. However, the most definitive reports so far indicate that:

- Only 1-5% of all colon cancers is linked statistically to genetic factors.[380]
- At most 2.5-10% of breast cancer cases may be genetically linked.[381]

Thus, we are back to WHO's estimate reported here earlier (Chapter 5) that 80% of all cancer occurrences are environmentally determined. If this is true, then perhaps 80% of the research effort needs to be directed toward combating environmentally related cancer. The argument for the link between heredity and cancer, at best, is that the cancer downstream has as its source the little pool upstream, known as the gene pool. This **assumption** leaves us with the analysis that: The abnormality upstream is the human condition – the human gene pool; and the human condition's gene pool is the reason for the debris of death and disease downstream.

A corollary to this assumption is that the individual is at fault for having "picked" the wrong parents; or, simply, that the family is at fault. Therefore, the victim is blamed. In any event, cancer-related genetic research appears to focus total attention upon one-factor that we can do absolutely nothing about, except slicing-off the breast of young women whose mothers, grandmothers, and older sisters have died of breast cancer.

Heredity-related cancer research may produce new insights into disease progression and even new advances in cancer therapy. However, genetically linked cancer research will not venture upstream far enough to staunch the flow. Genetically-based vision must climb out of its comfortable spot by the Gene Pool to observe what is going on in the fields beyond the fence and windbreak. Genetically-linked disease research of all kinds must consider the "interrelationship between genetic susceptibility and environmental exposures...."[382] Or, as Colburn and associates state it:

---

[380] G. Mara and C.R. Boland, "Hereditary Nonpolyposis Colorectal Cancer: The Syndrome, the Genes, and Historical Perspectives," Journal of the National Cancer Institute 87 (1995), 1114-1125

[381] G.A. Colditz, Family History, Age, and Risk of Breast Cancer: Prospective Data from the Nurses' Health Study, Journal of the American Medical Association 270 (1993), 338-343; See Watts, 28-29.

[382] Ibid.

The quest to discover the role of hormone-disrupting chemicals in… (breast and prostate cancer)deserves higher priority than the quest for hereditary breast and prostate cancer genes, because research aimed at environmental factors offers the hope of finding ways to prevent these devastating diseases in the vast majority of victims. [383]

The major corollary for the gene pool assumption noted above is that there is <u>nothing</u> we can do. That's just the way it is. People are going to get cancer. People are going to die of cancer. Plain and Simple However, Bruce Lipton, a cell biologist, makes the telling point that:

Even Darwin conceded, near the end of his life, that his evolutionary theory had shortchanged the role of environment. [384]

Lipton, then goes on to conclude:

In other words, when it comes to genetic control, 'It's the environment, stupid.' [385]

Julia Green Brody of the Silent Spring Institute is even more specific:

(Breast Cancer) incidence has stabilized in the U.S., but it's stabilized at one of the highest rates in the world and as women move from lower risk regions of the world to the U.S., their incidence goes up and continues to rise over a couple of generations. So we know that that's not genes and there's something about industrial society that's playing an important role. [386]

---

[383] <u>Our Stolen Future</u>, 186.

[384] Bruce Lipton, <u>The Biology of Belief: Unleashing the Power of Consciousness, Matter and Miracles</u>(Santa Rosa, CA: Authors Pub Corp, 2005), 50-where Lipton cites Darwin, F 1888.

[385] Ibid, 52.

[386] PCP 2010, 40.

Up and Down the Streams

The focus on genetic research tends to obscure the causes of cancer in the literal and real streams, rivers and creeks that run through our communities and croplands. To some extent it is true that for those who reside at the point of origin of stream pesticide pollution, there is no problem. For example, the Niobrara River has as its point of origin an innocent looking gurgle of water near Lusk, Wyoming. The Niobrara grows into an ever wider and more active stream as it courses eastward into Nebraska, being fed by numerous creeks. Ultimately, the Niobrara matures into a life-giving force for dozens of communities and hundreds of farms and ranches, thousands of people.

Any pesticide pollution, other than massive dumping of chemicals into the Niobrara near Lusk, would have little or no consequence to anyone living in all of Niobrara County, Wyoming, even the two communities downstream – Node and Van Tassel. In fact, there would be minimal consequence for the community of Marsland, Nebraska, 75 miles further downstream. Minimal consequence, that is, if the hypothetical pesticide pollution were the ONLY such incident. The fact is stream pollution in the Corn Belt states is rarely a function of a single source. Instead, as discussed throughout this book, the problem is a function of multiple occurrences leading to an accumulation of water toxicity.

The same process applies to:
- The West Nishnabotna River originating in the south west Iowa counties of Crawford, Carroll and Audubon with:
  + The West Fork forming directly south of Westside, Iowa; the East Fork emerging approximately seven miles north west of the town of Audubon; the main branch springing forth just to the south and east of Westside.
- The East Nishnabotna River taking shape at a source point in Carroll County very near the town of Templeton and approximately 12 miles north of Audubon.
- The Elkhorn River originating in north central Nebraska near the small town of Bassett in Rock County.
- The North Platte river originating in the west central Wyoming county of Natrona and whose stream flow is

> controlled at the Alcova Reservoir Dam south west of the city of Casper.
>
> - The South Platte originating in north west Colorado near the city of Greeley and whose stream flow is controlled at the Lake McConaughy Reservoir Dam in south west Nebraska near the city of Ogallala; and
> - The Rio Grande originating in central Colorado, fed by the Alamosa, Trihchera and Costilla rivers in Colorado; as well as numerous rivers in New Mexico, Texas, and Mexico before entering the Gulf of Mexico.

As the Nishnabotna, Elkhorn and Platte rivers flow to their ultimate convergences with the Missouri River, the level of toxicity increases at disproportionate and deadly rates due to the simple fact that the pesticides are extremely mobile in soil and lethally persistent in water.[387] Note for example that the USGS found ever increasing concentrations of atrazine in the North Platte as it flowed eastward from the city of North Platte, Nebraska, with an atrazine reading of .14ug/L, to Louisville, Nebraska, with a reading of .91ug/L (6.5 times the atrazine load accumulated in the 261 miles of river flow)[388]

The implications are deceiving. At first, it may seem that the problem of stream pollution decreases as one travels upstream. To an extent that is true – true only for those who reside upstream. However, if we use the example of the North Platte River, it is clear that as the river meanders its way from Alcova, Wyoming, to the Missouri River south of Omaha, the pollutant source-points are literally unknown in quantity.

What we do know is that the North Platte travels a total of 645 miles from Alcova, Wyoming, to the Missouri River in Nebraska, running through or skirting 86 towns and cities with a total population of 299,270 people.[389] Each home in these 86

---

[387] OPP, EPA (August 1999), 2.

[388] USGS, Water Quality in the Central Nebraska Basins: Major Issues and Findings,2.

[389] These statistics are, in part, taken from the State Farm Road Atlas (1997 Rand McNally, which are based on the 1990 census. Of the 86 towns and cities along the Platte considered here, 45 have no census data recorded in the State Farm document; therefore, population estimates for 1999 were utilized for 26 of those

communities is a potential polluter to the extent lawn and garden chemicals may be used.

In addition, there are the people living on ranches and farms along the river's course, and an untold number of gullies and drainage ditches that carry pesticides from soil runoff into the larger streams. We do know there are 108 creeks, canals, draws, and channels, sloughs and rivers that feed into the Platte River.[390]

Each one of the ranches and farms, each one of the gullies and drainage ditches, each one of the streams, creeks and rivers; each one of the families along the way, are potential source-points for endangerment of public health. Every one of the 299,270 people[391] is also a potential victim.

According to Safelawn Neighborhood Alliance, between 1989 and 1999 there was an astounding increase in the number of households nationally using chemicals on their lawns and gardens. Sixty-seven percent (67%) of American families are now using some form of pesticides to enhance their lawns and/or garden growth,[392] an increase from 55% a decade before.

Assuming a similar percentage of families are also using lawn and garden chemicals such as Roundup (glyphosate) in those communities along the Platte River, there would be 50,128 families practicing this form of weed and pest control. Assuming that each household annually utilizes a five-pound bag of such chemicals, we may estimate that between Alcova, Wyoming, and the confluence of the Platte and Missouri Rivers in southeastern Nebraska an additional 250,640 pounds of chemicals are applied to the soil within runoff range of the Platte. That means 389 pounds per mile and nearly one pound deposited every 14 feet,

Assuming, furthermore, that the chemical of choice for the inhabitants of the Platte River Valley matches the chemical of choice for the rest of the country and world, the 250,640 **pounds** of Roundup deposited along the Platte is but a miniscule amount

---

communities as available at: www.census.gov/population/estimates/metro-city/placebyst/SC99T7_NE.txt.

[390] EPA, "Surf Your Watershed."
www.cfpub.epa.gov/surf/locate/streamsperhuc_search.

[391] An estimate based on the assumption of 4 people/family.

[392] www.sit.wisc.edu/~safelawns.

compared to the 112,000 **tons** deposited world-wide in 1998.[393] Yet, the 250,640 pounds translates into an approximate total of 125 short tons. All of this so-called domestic use of pesticides is in addition to cropland pesticide use and consequent runoff into ground and surface waters.

One might argue that many householders anxious to have the greenest lawns and the most productive gardens do not know how best to apply roundup or any other chemical. Therefore, the argument may take us to requiring licensed/certified applicators for all chemicals and requiring the establishment of a "Pesticide Sensitive Registry" in every state and community.[394] But the fact remains that pesticides are still being applied to the land worldwide, and those chemicals are extremely toxic, including "wartime defoliants such as Agent Orange, nerve-gas type pesticides, and artificial hormones."[395]

One might also argue that the folks of Rural Small-Town America, and the corn belt in particular, would be less likely to afford the expenditures required to apply Roundup or any other chemicals. They would certainly be unlikely customers of companies such as True Green (formerly ChemLawn). To an extent such an argument holds its own. But the argument loses its force the closer one moves toward a river's shores.

---

[393] "New Study Links Monsanto's Roundup to Cancer," (June 1999) www.biotech-info.net/glyphosate_cancer.

[394] As of March 1999, eight states (Colorado, Connecticut, Florida, Maryland, Michigan, Pennsylvania, Washington, and West Virginia) had legislated the establishment of local Pesticide Sensitive Registries. The average number of people with chemical sensitivities registering ranged from 8.2 million in Michigan to 66.6 million in Florida. See Dr. Catherine Daniela, Pesticide Coordinator, WSU, Pesticide Sensitive Registry in Washington and Other States. www.tricity.wsu.edu/aenews/Mar99AENews.
By 2003 eleven states (Louisiana, Maine and Wisconsin in addition to the 8 noted previously) had established such registries. See: www.dhh.Louisiana.gov/offices/publications/pubs-05/FINALHypersensitivityRegistry. (No update available as of October 10, 2018.)

[395] Chris Syrengelas, "Lawn Pesticides," Interdisciplinary Minor in Global Sustainability, Senior Seminar (Irvine: University of California, 1997). www.mamba.bio.uci.edu/~pjbryant/global/sen_sem/syren97.

Riverfront and river view property, no matter where one goes, is most expensive. Only the wealthier among us can afford to purchase and keep up with the annual taxes on such land. The wealthier river site owners are also those who are most likely to subscribe to the services of companies such as True Green. Therefore, it would be no surprise to learn that riverfront and river-view landowners are the most inclined to apply chemicals to their lawns and gardens.

Problem of Problems: Bio-Magnification

While the symptoms of high rates of cancer may occur the further downstream we go, the fact is the causes lie upstream. It is like a flood is happening all around us and we do not see it. The Problem of Problems, we might say, began upstream when:

- the first farmer or rancher used DDT or atrazine,
- or when the first homeowner/gardener applied Roundup or Diazinon;
- or when the first crop was dusted from the air;
- or when the first central pivot began the steady process of washing simazine off the land into the ditches and gullies destined for creeks, rivers, and lakes;
- or when the first central pivot doubled its efficiency by spraying pesticides as well as water;
- or when the first central pivot chemigator "hiccupped" and siphoned the pesticides into the family's and/or community's water supply.

The Problem of Problems continues with each repeated application of all-of-the-above, and more. The Problem of Problems in a word is **Bio-Magnification** – the process whereby the larger organisms along the food chain absorb the higher concentrations of all things ingested, higher concentrations of the good as well as the bad. Larger fish absorb higher concentrations of protean as well as higher concentrations of pesticides. Cows and horses absorb more of the same than do rabbits or birds. Adult humans absorb more nutritional elements than do children. Unfortunately, nursing mothers pass along high concentrations of pesticides in their breast milk as well.[396]

But the burning question is this: Given all that has been discussed so far, where do we go from here?

---

[396] Steingraber # 1, 168, 192, 222. See also, "Biomagnification: how DDT becomes concentrated as it passes through the food chain," www.users.ren.com/jkimball.ma.ultranet/BiologyPages/D/DDTandTrophicLevel, (8 August 2003): From Biology (Wm. C. Brown, 1994) by Dr. John Kimball.

Chapter Twelve:

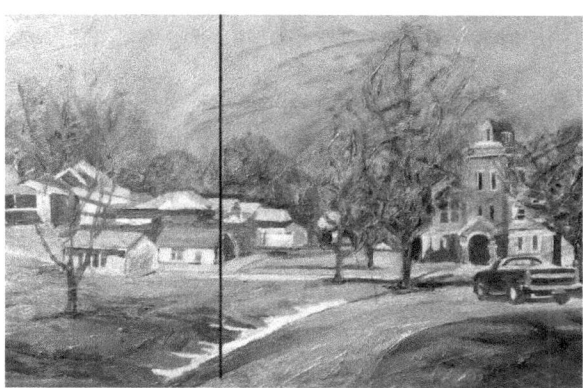

County Courthouse

Toward the End of Victimization:
Where Do We Go from Here?

<u>Victimization</u>

Lieutenant/Farmer Duane was able to articulate the belief that Agent Orange had made him a victim and casualty of the Vietnam War. Duane firmly believed he was an American Victim of that war in every sense of the word. He spoke out and charged his own country with his pending death.

Most of the women presented here expressed, as noted repeatedly, the question of "what did I do wrong?" In so doing they were articulating a readiness to accept blame for their own illnesses.

Just by raising the question of what they may have done "wrong," Donna Jo and others betrayed a readiness to be victimized a second time by believing their terminal diagnosis of cancer was somehow their own fault. These women were ready to accept guilt, comparable to the guilt often heaped upon a rape victim. Society often indicts the rape victim for having worn the wrong clothes or having been in the wrong place. Thus, the rape is the victim's own fault, and the victim is victimized all over again. In the case of cancer, victims are often "accused" of having the wrong parents, the wrong set of genes, leading the wrong lifestyles, or just being stubborn and staying put by refusing to leave.

The victims of cancer have a great deal of help in accepting guilt. The chemical companies and those who defend them "typically blame the victims, deny the problem, and try to avoid responsibility for the harm caused."[397] On the other hand, the chemical industry has been known to acknowledge that their chemicals have indeed resulted in even the contamination of human breast milk. The corporate "solution," however, is to urge mothers to stop breast feeding. The real solution is totally ignored by the chemical industry, their lobbyists, and other enablers: namely: *Stop the contamination of breast milk in the first place.*[398]

So, what can we really do? This chapter addresses that very question in the context of finding models for action.

Where Do We Go from Here?

Rather than 'use' our resources, we are challenged to transform them. Just as in some religious mystery…we must, in solving the problem, solve ourselves… Mystery appears in many guises:
- *as the disease that defies cure,*
- *as the faltering institutional system,*
- *as the ineffective ideology,*
- *as the persistent sense of failed opportunity.*
  (Robert Grudin)[399]

The "mystery" that resides at the center of this book seems to qualify on every one of philosopher Robert Grudin's criteria:
- Cancer is a *disease that defies cure,*
- Government (local, state, regional, and national) is a *faltering institutional system,*
- American agricultural, scientific, military, economic, and social policies are all a piece of a most *ineffective ideology.*

---

[397] Ann McCampbell, MD, "Multiple Chemical Sensitivity Under Siege."
[398] Watts, 140.
[399] Robert Grudin, The Grace of Great Things – Creativity and Innovation (Ticknor and Fields, 1990), 44-45.

- Taking the long-view, we can see, understand, and feel the *persistent sense of failed opportunity* to prevent and stop the suffering upon and to American soil, as well as the soil of nearly every nation in this world of ours. For example, one in eight of every American women run the risk of having to combat breast cancer. Unless we stop the madness, "most of their daughters and all of **their** (emphasis added) daughters (will) develop the disease. Such a future is unacceptable."[400]

In some countries, as reported by Watts of New Zealand, the situation is immensely dire. In Malaysia and elsewhere, women constitute as much or more than "85% of the pesticide applicators on commercial farms and plantations, often working whilst pregnant or breast-feeding. There are an estimated 30,000 women pesticide sprayers in Malaysia alone. They spray pesticides…on average 262 days per year."[401]

As the President's Cancer Panel notes:

Approximately 41 percent of Americans will be diagnosed with cancer at some point in their lives and about 21 percent will die from cancer.[402]

But what can we do? In fact, is there no other way? Are the generations to come doomed to suffer the consequences of this generation's actions, obsessions, and inactions? Let us consider the possibilities:

Gourds & Purple Martins: A Cherokee Lesson

---

[400] Andrea Martin, "Reclaiming Our Birthright," Silent Spring Review Fall 2000, 12.
[401] Watts, 10; citing Joshi, Fernandez, Mourin, and Pengam, Poisoned & Silenced: A Study of Pesticide Poisoning in the Plantations (Tenganita, PAN, Penang, 2002).
[402] PCP 2010, Executive Summary, I.

The Cherokee Nation had it figured out a long time ago. Long before the White Man invented pesticides to keep plant-eating creatures of nature away from eating his crops, the Cherokee knew of a better and more sustainable way. They kept the "pests" away from their corn crops, their life-sustaining corn, by simply hanging gourds from poles around the fields. The gourds, they knew, would attract Purple Martins who nest and establish primacy of turf over any other bird that might venture forth onto the sacred cropland – sacred to both Bird and Men & Women. The Purple Martin would fight the corn-eating Crow away. The Purple Martin fed voraciously upon the insects foolish enough to invade this protected property.

The result? The Purple Martin prospered, as they "fought the good fight" for themselves and for the Cherokee who provided the Martin with "Landing Rights" and respect. The Crow and Insect learned to go elsewhere, or they paid the price. The Cherokee prospered.

We have much to learn from the Cherokee. They did not look to deadlier and deadlier ways to poison the things of creation that were inconvenient or even threatening their way of life. The Cherokee possess a cosmology that opens doors to understanding nature, nurture, and survival.

According to the Cherokee Creation Story, it was the Water Beetle who volunteered to venture above the ocean to see if there was something beyond the water world itself. As he came to the surface, all he saw was water. So, he decided to go to the very bottom of the ocean floor. From there the Water Beetle scooped up and carried to the surface of the ocean a huge cache of mud. The Water Beetle's labor paid off almost immediately as the mud became transformed into an island. From the island, trees soon began to grow and a whole new world of existence was now available to the ocean creatures. Then came bird and animal life.

One day, lightning hit a tree on the island. The tree caught fire. The creatures knew there was a power in fire. If only they could use it. First the Raven tried to fly into the fire and bring some of it out for all to use. The fire was too hot, and that is why the Raven is black. The Owl tried to do the same, but he had to retreat. The fire and smoke were too much for his wide eyes to bear. That is why, after rubbing and rubbing his eyes, that the Owl has big eyes and can bear to venture forth only at night.

Finally, it was the Water Beetle who came through for the second time. He formed a bowl from the mud, carried it under the burning tree, and caught some fire in the bowl, and brought the bowl and fire out. And that is how the Cherokee came to have the power of fire.

Creation, Cosmology & Theology

And THAT is how the Cherokee, the Fire People, possess a profound understanding of creation that far surpasses the Judeo-Christian perspective. The Cherokee know that their very existence has, from the beginning, depended upon even the smallest of the Great Spirit's creatures. Because of all that the Water Beetle did, the Cherokee have the greatest respect, as well, for all of the Water Beetle's insect relatives. Thus, the Fire People instinctively "go with the flow" of the inter-connectedness of life. Rather than pursuing a "slash and burn" approach to solving a problem between the forces of Nature and their goal of survival, they adapt their understanding of how Nature functions to defining the means to achieve their goals. So it is that the Fire People use Nature to nurture themselves.[403]

The Judeo-Christian perspective may find in the Book of Genesis the justification, even a perverted sense of a sacred call, to subject all of creation to human purposes. Unfortunately, this view of Creation boxes everything into neat and separate categories: the land, the sea, the animals, the birds, the fish, and finally the human. Then God rested and said it was good. God then gave the human dominion over the whole thing. Indeed, as Susan Power Bratton laments while referencing Genesis 1:27:

To use creation in God's image as an excuse for environmental destruction is to despiritualize the text and miss the point.[404]

When the notion of dominion is combined with God's call to exercise power over the land, the sea, and the air, we have a deadly

---

[403] The Cherokee Story of Creation is recounted here as told at the Museum of the Cherokee Indian, Cherokee, North Carolina (October 2001).
[404] Susan Power Bratton, Christianity, Wilderness, and Wildlife: The Original Desert Solitaire (Scranton, PA: University of Scranton Press, 1993), 292.

Cosmology – a cosmology that authorizes eliminating anything and everything that stands in our way. The Cherokee know differently. The Cherokee Way is the way of sustainability. It is instructive to note that the American Catholic Bishops have called us to listen to the Cherokee and other native/indigenous peoples:

Many indigenous technologies can teach us much. Such technologies are compatible with the ecosystem, are much more available to poor persons, and are more sustainable for the entire community. [405]

Sustainable Agriculture – A Paradigm Shift

Industrial agriculture is devastating our land, water, and our air, and is now threatening the sustainability of the biosphere. Its massive chemical and biological inputs cause widespread environmental havoc as well as human disease and death.

Its monoculturing reduces the diversity of our plants and animals. Its habitat destruction endangers wildlife. Its Factory-farming practices cause untold animal suffering. Its centralized corporate ownership destroys farm communities…leading to mass poverty and hunger.

The industrial agricultural system is clearly unsustainable. It has truly become a fatal harvest.
(Andrew Kimbrel) [406]

Upstream solutions to the downstream glut of cancer problems would certainly include re-acquainting ourselves with the ancient wisdom of traditional peoples and the "new" concept of sustainable agriculture. "Sustainable" derives from the Latin "sustinere" – "to hold up." To practice "sustainable Agriculture" is to engage in "food

---

[405] National Conference of Catholic Bishops, <u>Renewing the Earth: An Invitation to Reflection and Action on Environment in Light of Catholic Social Teaching – A Pastoral Statement of the United States Catholic Conference.</u> (November 14, 1991, IVB.)
[406] Kimbrel, 3.

production practices that can be 'kept up' or 'held up' for the length of time that human beings will need food."[407]

In the early 1970s many Nebraska farmers became interested in organic farming because they had concluded that so-called conventional farming was on a dead-end street. As these farmers viewed the matter:

- Conventional agriculture was too reliant on costly chemicals.
- They were seeing poor crop yields even with the chemicals that were annually increasing in cost while crop prices were annually decreasing.
- They had become increasingly doubtful about the long-term effectiveness of the agrichemicals, especially pesticides.
- They had grown fearful of the effect of the chemicals upon their health, the health of their families, the health of their livestock, and the health of the land.[408]

After the completion of a government-sponsored study of the Talwandi Sabo block, Bathinda District, Punjab, India, Dr. S.G. Kabra, a senior environmentalist with the Indian Institute of Health Management and Research, concluded:

The report is a clear indication towards the fact that Punjab needs to be freed from the clutches of pesticides immediately. The extensive use of pesticides in (the) cotton belt is spelling doom not only for flora but for fauna as well.[409]

Perhaps Pope Francis states it best in what he claims is his major appeal:

The urgent challenge to protect our common home includes a concern to bring the whole human family together to seek a sustainable and integral development....[410]

---

[407] Sustainable Agriculture in Nebraska: A Status Report, by Mary Bruns (Walthill, Nebraska: Center for Rural Affairs, November 1986), 1.
[408] Ibid, 4.
[409] Mega Mohan.
[410] Pope Francis, 13.

A Consideration of the Alternatives

Perhaps the major alternative to "conventional" farming, gardening, and lawn care is to adopt a different paradigm – a paradigm of cooperating with Nature rather than trying to subdue Her. As Mark Winston defines the problem:

The most important effect of our chosen role in nature as dominators rather than as stewards has been to lose our sense of place in the biological world around us.[411]

Well over 100 years ago Liberty Hyde Bailey counseled those who would listen that we must learn to "live in right relationship" with the environment in which we live.[412] To switch roles from subduer to cooperator is not an easy task.

The old cliché, "you can't teach old dogs new tricks," is certainly part of the hurdle. For one thing, continuing with past practice is simply easier: we do not need to expend energy in becoming acquainted with the new. Secondly, the new may even produce less attractive produce; the apples and pears, corn and cabbage may be more uneven in appearance, quality and availability to the consumer.[413] What would be sacrificed, however, is the god of convenience rather than continuing to sacrifice human lives to and for that same god.

Sustainable agriculture, while being most organic and holistic in approach, is not necessarily organic farming. Organic farming is one approach to sustainable agriculture. Sustainable agriculture is a philosophy and "a goal rather than a rigidly defined set of practices."[414] The goals of sustainable agriculture are economic and environmental. The farm must provide adequate production to meet

---

[411] Mark L. Winston, <u>Nature Wars: People vs. Pests</u> (Cambridge: Harvard University Press, 1997), 174.

[412] Wes Jackson, "Farming in Nature's Image: Natural Systems Agriculture," in Kimbrel, 72, citing Bailey's 1915 book, <u>The Holy Earth</u>.

[413] Canadian Network, 12-13.

[414] <u>A Better Row to Hoe: The Economic, Environmental, and Social Impact of Sustainable Agriculture</u> (St. Paul, Minnesota: Northwest Area Foundation, December 1994), 2.

economic needs of the farm family, but at the same time the means to that end are determined with an eye to maintaining the integrity of the farmland's natural environment. Sustainable farmers wrestle with maximizing production, while also maximizing ecological strategies, as well as diminishing reliance on chemicals and non-renewable energy resources.

Sustainable farming requires a shift in the agricultural paradigm. Sustainability brings with it a genuine respect for the land as a non-expendable resource. Conventional farming looks to production first with sustainability of the land a distant alternative concern (if at all). Conventional farming tends to seek the maximum yield to be taken from the land. Sustainable agriculture seeks a balance between taking from and giving back. Conventional farming tends to concentrate on one or two crops, while sustainable farming practices the art and science of diversification.

Michael Pollan outlines in his book, The Omnivore's Dilemma: A Natural History of Four Meals, a helpful comparative description of the differences between a so-called Conventional Farm operation and a Sustainable Farm: The Conventional Farm vs. the Polyface Farm. The former typology is based on a north central Iowa farm where Pollan had spent time working with the farmer. The latter typology is based on a western Virginia (as opposed to West Virginia) farm operation. The difference in style of farming may be generalized, in part as follows:

Conventional Farming	vs.	**Sustainable Farming**
*Industrial Technique & Philosophy		Pastoral Technique & Philosophy
*Annual species cultivated		Perennial species cultivated
*Single-crop focused		Multi/diversified crops
*Fossil energy dependent		Solar energy to extent possible
*Global market targeted		Local market exclusively
*Mechanical		Biological[415]

In a study of Midwestern agriculture conducted by the Northwestern Area foundation (NAF) in 1989, it was found that sustainable farmers in Iowa used two-thirds less pesticides and three-

---

[415] Michael Pollan, Omnivore's Dilemma: A Natural History of Four Meals (Penguin Press, 2006, 130-131), Typology adapted.

fourths les synthetic fertilizers as compared to conventional farmers.[416] Let it be noted, however, that farmers like Joel Salatin and his Polyface Farm use absolutely no pesticides or synthetic fertilizers, and their farms thrive.[417] The NAF study also noted that Sustainable farmers had more crops in production, relied significantly less on corn for revenue, and their soil and corn tested markedly lower for nitrate content than was the case for conventional farms.

Furthermore, sustainable farms had over three times as much land held in "non-productive" use such as protecting wetlands.[418] Expanding the size and number of wetlands in the Midwest is believed to be one of the most sustainable solutions to the Dead Zone hundreds of miles downstream from the origins of the Platte, Elkhorn, Niobrara and Nishnabotna Rivers.

The Midwest has sacrificed approximately 80% of its wetland to industrialized agriculture over the course of the last two centuries, compared to a 50% loss elsewhere in the continental United States. Although nearly 577,000 acres of wetlands have already been recreated, anywhere from 5,700,000 to 14,425,000 acres of additional wetlands need to be created or restored in order to detoxify the Gulf of Mexico.[419] Less than one year before the September 2005 Hurricane Katrina devastated New Orleans, the Philadelphia Inquirer warned that because "1,900 square mils of Louisiana wetlands, an area the size of Delaware, have been lost since 1930," New Orleans, especially was considered vulnerable to "becoming another Atlantis..."[420] In other words, the practice of sustainable agriculture provides a benefit not only for the individual

---

[416] "The Northwest Area Foundation is committed to helping reduce poverty for the long term in rural, urban, American Indian, and rural Latino communities in Minnesota, Iowa, North Dakota, South Dakota, Montana, Idaho, Washington, and Oregon." Northwest Area foundation. www.nwaf.org/About.
[417] Pollan, Omnivore's Dilemma, 123-273.
[418] Ibid, 5-8.
[419] "More Information on the 'Dead Zone.'" www.earthsky.com/2001/esmi011127.
[420] Paul Nussbaum, "New Orleans' growing danger: Wetlands loss leaves city a hurricane hit away from disaster," (Philadelphia Inquirer, October 8, 2004) www.hurricane.lsu.edu/_in_the_news/phillyinquirer100804.

farmer, but also for the neighborhood, the state, the region, and all of creation downstream.[421]

Sustainability is not just a farming issue, it is an issue for all urban and rural dwellers. Sustainability as a homeowner with a lawn or garden to care for, means doing things differently. By such action, we contribute to an important decline in what the land and our neighbor have been forced to endure. Instead of the greenest lawn in town, how about a switch to more natural lawns with native grasses, rocks and stones, bushes and shrubs, or raised garden that require little maintenance and no pesticides or nitrates?

Hudson, Quebec, a suburb of Montreal, exercising the Precautionary Principle, banned the use of lawn pesticides in 1991. From 1991 to 2001 thirty-six other Quebec towns enacted similar ordinances. Similar laws have been enacted in six other provinces as well as two of the three Arctic territories.[422] Communities in the U.S., such as Lawrence, Kansas, have followed suit.[423]

These policies can impact what is, in fact, our largest crop:

America's biggest crop is not corn, wheat, or soy beans. It is 'turfgrass' – the stuff lawns are made of. The crop in question covers some 25 million acres, or four thousand square miles, which is just a shade less than the area of Pennsylvania... The average acre of American lawn gets four times as much pesticide as the average acre of farmland.[424]

---

[421] See also Oran B. Hesterman, Ph.D, Fair Food: Growing A Healthy, Sustainable Food System for All (NY: Public Affairs, 2011) for discussion of other alternatives including: "Ridge-Till" (79) and "Integrated Pest Management" (106).

[422] "Canadian Supreme Court Rules in Favor of Residential Pesticide Ban," Beyond Pesticides Daily News Archive, July 7, 2001. www.beyondpesticides.org/NEWS/daily_news_archive/07_02_01.html.

[423] John Kepner, "Around the Country," Pesticides and You (Vol 22, No. 3, 2003).

[424] Evan Eisenberg, The Ecology of Eden (Alfred Knopf, 1998), 251-253.

Intensify Multiple Chemical Exposure Research:
The Call for A Cancer Early Warning System

Serious research regarding MCE must include its possible linkage with chemically induced cancer. Would a close and intense study of MCE symptoms lead to a better understanding of the early symptoms of cancer? Could such a study lead to a Cancer Early Warning System (CEWS)? If such studies were done, could it have made a difference in the lives of Donna Jo, Susan, Sandra, JoAn, Shelley, Helen and Ben, and Duane?

MCE is a poorly understood and under-investigated area, both in terms of on-going research and enforcement of exposure limitation standards. As pointed out in Chapter Four, MCE research is stunted due to the nature of the beast, i.e., where do you start and where do you stop. Scientific research is frustrated by the proliferation of possible exposures to carcinogens. But one thing is clear: funding from the chemical industry to conduct the research is hardly a reliable and safe answer.

While the establishment of Pesticide Sensitivity Registries (PSRs) is a start, they are, in and of themselves, a minor preventative. PSRs must be given more enforcement teeth than is currently the case. PSRs, as we know them in 11 states that have such laws, are merely public notification laws with limited application. A person who registers with PSR must be diagnosed with a Multiple Chemical Sensitivity (MCS). There are countless numbers of people with MCS who do not know it. But even if they do get to register, so what? All it means is that a pesticide applicator must give prior notification that a pesticide will be applied on a date certain. PSRs have no power to halt such applications.

If PSRs are to have any meaning at all, if PSRs are to make any difference in the wanton destruction of human life and spoilage of the land, then the presence of one person so registered and living in a reasonable contiguous area must require the prohibition of pesticide application. To do otherwise is to say that even one person's life is expendable. Zero Tolerance must become policy; and, as discussed in Chapter Four, a zero tolerance of Maximum Contaminant Levels must become enforceable policy rather than simply a desirable and flexible goal. At present, any MCL is only a feeble suggestion.

Zero Tolerance, the Precautionary Principle, and the Least Toxic Alternative may be keys to bringing wholeness back to the land and its people. However, perhaps the real key to ending this Tragedy lies in the education and re-education of us all, especially the education that occurs through one's experience of the "Pilot's Dilemma."

The Pilot's Dilemma, Our Challenge

Andrew Kimbrel recounts[425] seeing the stage play, The Rescue, concerning an American pilot shot down over North Vietnam. The pilot is rescued and protected by a farmer. Over time, the pilot falls in love with the farmer's daughter. Life goes reasonably well for a while, until one-day when a contingent of American Green Berets arrive to "rescue" the pilot. However, the commandos insist that they must kill the farmer and his daughter, both of whom are now security risks. Failing in his efforts to reason with the Green Berets, the pilot solves his dilemma by shooting himself.

The point is that the pilot had no problem dropping his load of bombs from a distance of 30,000 feet, slaughtering untold numbers of people; but once he came face-to-face with what he once considered the enemy, developing relationships with them as human beings, "he would rather kill himself than cause their deaths."

The point of the Pilot's Dilemma here is that perhaps what it will take for us all to fathom the enormity of what we are doing to our own families, our neighbors, and our very selves with our chemical dependency, is to come face-to-face with how the enemy is us. Then there will be more public support for sustainable agriculture, sustainable living, organic farming, and financing for alternatives to pesticides.

---

[425] Andrew Kimbrel, "Organic and Beyond," (Bioneers Letter, Autumn 2003), 11-12.

Human Rights & Sustainability

All of us who eat have to become conscientious objectors to the war against nature.[426]

For significant change to occur, before we completely desecrate the land, the planet, and ourselves, it will take a form of activism, specifically a Human Rights approach. A human rights response to the deleterious effects of pesticides on human health, according to Sandra Steingraber, "recognizes that the current system of regulating the use, release, and disposal of known and suspected carcinogens – rather than preventing their generation in the first place – is intolerable."[427]

A human rights perspective leading to political action would acknowledge that the present regulatory routines and apparatus operate in a context of "reckless disregard for human life."[428] Indeed, when cancer-causing chemicals are released into the environment, "some number of vulnerable persons are consigned to death. The impossibility of tabulating an exact body count does not alter this fact."[429]

A human rights stance in fighting for a cleaner, safer and saner environment understand that on one point those who lobby for and against the chemical industry agree:

A certain level of risk must always be associated with human exposure to any chemical.[430]

Indeed, even Rachel Carson, as much as she warned of the hazards of DDT, never advocated for the elimination of all

---

[426] Ron Kroese, "Industrial Agriculture's War Against Nature," in Kimbrel, The Fatal Harvest, 105.

[427] Steingraber #1, 268; #2, 280.

[428] Ibid.

[429] Ibid.

[430] C.F. Wilkinson, "The Science and Politics of Pesticides," in Silent Spring Revisited, 40. Note that Wilkinson's point is accompanied by the realization that the limits of science make it so. Wilkinson's leanings are toward a lightening-up on the regulation of the chemical industry. Sandra Steingraber makes the same point in her call for even stricter regulation of chemicals to extent of elimination.

chemicals, taking the position that if used properly chemicals can be beneficial to humankind.[431]

Yet, it took 24 years for the EPA to issue a Registration Standard for atrazine, after it had been used widely. Twenty-nine years after atrazine's introduction into the environment, EPA issued a "preliminary notification" of intent to conduct a "Special Review…based on carcinogenic potential and possible risks resulting from exposure through the diet from treated food and contaminated water, as well as concerns of potential carcinogenic risk to pesticide mixers and applicators."[432] Thirty-one years and thousands of tons later, EPA classified atrazine in 1990 as a "Restricted Use Pesticide." Thirty-five years had then passed before EPA found reason in 1994 to caution that atrazine exposure "through food and water, through the use of lawn care products, and by occupational exposures in pesticide applicators, may 'pose risks of concern.'"[433]

Note that after the World Trade Center was destroyed in 2001 and we learned that Middle Eastern hijackers of the planes had trained in American flight schools, we did not wait until 2030 to issue a "preliminary notification" of intent to conduct a "Special Review" of the matter. Furthermore, we did not plan to wait until 2040 to decide on the level of acceptable risk. Action was taken immediately to deal with the perceived risk. Yet, in the case of the terror that reigns over public health due to the threat of tens of thousands of domestic chemicals, only 450 had been tested as of 1999 by the National Toxicology Program for their relationship to breast cancer.[434] Eleven years later (2010), the President's Cancer Panel reported:

Only a few hundred of the more than 80,000 chemicals in use in the U.S. have been tested for safety.[435]

---

[431] A point made repeatedly in Souder.

[432] BCERF, "Critical Evaluation," 3.

[433] Ibid, 4.

[434] Susan S. Ballis, "Did the Environment Cause My Breast Cancer?" <u>Silent Spring Review</u>, (Summer 1999), 9.

[435] PCP, 2010, ii.

But only 3 years had passed before it could be reported that the situation had become even more dire. As of April 2013, while the latest version of the "Safe Chemicals Act" was being considered by the US Senate, Paragraph 2 made the claim that:

More than 84,000 chemicals are on the Environmental Protection Agency's inventory…and an average of 700 new chemicals are introduced each year.[436]

This writer endorses the viewpoint expressed by Peter Montague that:

Murder is murder even if the victim is anonymous. And scientists, risk assessors, and regulators who grease the wheels for such a system – even if only by complicit silence – have blood on their hands. They are the enablers of a system that profoundly violates the human rights of the thousands (or millions) whom it victimizes.[437]

It took Rosa Parks to put her foot down and say, "No more!" One woman stood up to authority. One woman stood up against the way things were and always had been. One woman stood up to the way the world was, and said, "I'm tired of it!" One woman sat down in a front seat refusing to sit in the back, tagging along behind where other people were going. One woman stood out from all others and sparked the fire of the US Civil Rights Movement. This same woman died of cancer – one of 7.6 million others who die of cancer each year worldwide.[438]

Rosa Parks died of a disease as discriminatory as the social disease of racial discrimination. Having been raised on a farm near Montgomery, Alabama[439] and most likely having worked in the

---

[436] https://www.gov/track.us/congress/bills/113/s696/text. See also, Ian Urbina, "Think Those Chemicals Have Been Tested?" The New York Times (April 13, 2013 www.nytimes.com/2013/04/14/Sinday-review/think-those-chemical-have-been-tested.

[437] Peter Montague, "Living Downstream – a review," Rachel's Environment & Health Weekly #565, September 25, 1997. www.pmac.net/downstream, 4.

[438] CDC, "World Cancer Day." www.cdc.gov/features/worldcancerday.

[439] Academy of Achievement, "Rosa Parks Biography: Pioneer of Civil Rights," (October 31, 2005) www.achievement.org/autodoc/page/parObio-1.

cotton fields as a young girl, she may well have died from causes that could easily have been avoided and situations over which she had no control.

It is long overdue for us to hear the pleas of a woman who at the time of writing her book was dying of cancer, Rachel Carson. Her plea to the US Congress, echoing back to us from 50 years ago, that we give full respect to:

The right of the citizen to be secure in his own home against the intrusion of poisons applied by other persons ... should be one of the basic human rights.[440]

Indeed, Pope Francis forcefully puts forth the notion that:

Access to safe drinkable water is a basic and universal human right, since it is essential to human survival and, as such, is a condition for the exercise of other human rights.[441]

Perhaps it will take a Rosa Parks to sit-in at a pesticide plant, or sit-in on the middle of field about to be sprayed with pesticides, or set up a booth at the local county fair serving free coffee, free tea, free Kool-Aid, free concentrated fruit juices and served up with water officially certified as "safe" by a mere .01 MCL according to EPA's "safe" standards, but of course with the appropriate disclosures and requiring that each customer sign a waiver of responsibility for any resulting illness from drinking the liquid of their choice.

We need to learn from those in Argentina who have taken a stand against the Monsanto Corporation. For six months residents of the town of Malvinas, Province of Cordoba, blockaded the site where Monsanto was constructing what would have become the "world's largest maize seed treatment plant."[442] By maintaining at least a 200

---

[440] Cited by Julia G. Brody, Silent Spring Review (Winter 2002), 2.

[441] Pope Francis, 30.

[442] Fabiana Frayssinet, "Argentina Activists Win First Round Against Monsanto Plant," http://www,nationofchange.org. See also: * Michael Warren and Natacha Pisarenko, "Argentines link health problems to agrochemicals," http://www.kob.com/article/stories/S3197070, and * Erin Gallagher, "Malvinas

day vigil, including keeping 30 tents staked to the entrance to Monsanto's project, the protesters won a court order to stop construction until an environmental assessment would be conducted and public hearings held. They took a stand and made their point. By March 2016 Monsanto's website no longer even mentioned the project, and by April 2017 Monsanto had sold the property to Regam/AMG.[443] The property remains vacant as of this writing (October 11, 2018).

Also, there is the example offered by Haitian farmers on Easter Day 2010. They communicated their opinion of a "generous" gift by Monsanto to Haiti in the wake of a devastating earthquake. On that day the farmers of Haiti gathered to receive Monsanto's "grand gift" of "sixty thousand bags of sterile seeds. These seeds, known as terminator seeds, would have required the farmers "to buy herbicides, pesticides and other poisons from the genetically modified pharmacy." Instead these Haitian farmers "burned every sack in an immense bonfire."[444]

In the U.S., being a litigious country, there have been numerous lawsuits filed and fought regarding the USEPA's action and in-actions. Among those initiating such action are: *Beyond Pesticides, The Center for Biological Diversity, The Center for Food Safety, Earth Justice, The Environmental Working Group, The National Family Farm Coalition, The National Resource Defense Council, and The Pesticide Action Network, North America.*

While the legal work of these, and other, organizations has certainly had an effect in terms of holding the EPA to its mandates, and raising public awareness, perhaps a 2011 Supreme Court decision may offer the basis for effective legal means of overturning the power and influence of all chemical companies in the U.S.:

Argentina: 200 Day Blockade Against Monsanto," Revolution News, April 5, 2014 http://revolution-nedws.com/malvinas-argentina-200-day-blockade-monsanto. All accessed March 20, 2015.

[443] LAVOZ Editorial Staff, "Socio-environmental conflicts: Monsanto in Malvinas, a badge," (April 23, 2017) http://www.lavoz.com.ar/loultimo.

[444] "Suicide Seeds," Eduardo Galeano, Children of the Days: A Calendar of Human History (NY: Nation Books, 2013), 250.

Raising the Stakes for Corporate Data Manipulation:
Enter the Stake Holder

Background

On May 22, 2011, the U.S. Supreme Court handed down a decision which may open the door to litigation against chemical companies not available until now. The case before the Court was that of MATRIXX INITIATIVES., ER AL. v. SIRACUSANO ER AL. (No. 09-1156).[445]

At first glance, Matrixx v. Siracusano (to be referred to hereafter as Matrixx) might appear to have little to do with pesticides. Afterall, Matrixx is a pharmaceutical company sued by investors in its product, a cold remedy marketed as Zicam. At issue were the following claims:

- The investors (Siracusano, et al) alleged that Matrixx knowingly withheld vital information from them; namely, reports and studies indicating harmful effects from the use of Zicam, i.e., the loss of the sense of smell (anosimia). In legal terms Siracusano alleged that Matrixx committed *Scienter*, the act of knowingly and deliberately withholding vital information.[446]
- Matrixx countered that it did not withhold vital information because there was none to share. This defense was based on the position that there was no statistically significant studies or reports indicating that Zicam caused the loss of smell. In other words, Matrixx claimed that no studies existed that would be of material interest to investors of the courts, and that all the plaintiffs were concerned with was anecdotal in nature. In this instance Matrixx put forth the legal defense of the *Bright-Line Rule,* that proof-positive evidence must be presented by plaintiffs. Siracusano, of course argued in opposition to Mattrixx's brief.

---

[445] Matrixx Initiatives, Inc., et al. v. Siracusano et. Al. Certiorari to the United States Court of Appeals for the Ninth Circuit. No. 09-1156. Argued January 10, 2011 – Decided March 22, 2011 www.supremecourt.gov.
[446] Syllabus, 2.

The Supreme Court ruled 9-0 against Matrixx with Justice Sonya Sotomayor writing the opinion. The major points of law issued by the Court are as follow:

- The bright-line rule does not apply.
- Statistically significant data is not necessary, nor is it the only relevant and material information.
- Matrixx failed the test of scienter.

In laymen's terms the Supreme Court of the United States ruled 9-0 that this pharmaceutical company lied and manipulated information with the intent to deceive investors and potential investors in its product.

The Court noted:

Matrixx's premise that statistical significance is the only reliable indication of causation is flawed. Both medical experts and the Food and Drug Administration rely on evidence other than statistically significant data to establish an inference of causation. It thus stands to reason that reasonable investors would act on such evidence.

In addition, the Court ruled that while:

Something more than the mere existence of adverse reports…that something more is not limited to statistical significance and can come from the source, content, and context of the reports.[447]

Furthermore, it was held that Matrixx had:

Received reports from medical experts and researchers that plausibly indicated a reliable causal link between Zicam and anosimia.

Therefore, the Court went on to charge Matrixx with failing its own invocation of the bright-line rule in that it:

---

[447] Loc cit.

Elected not to disclose adverse event reports not because it believed that they were meaningless but because it understood their likely effect on the market.[448]

In fact, in the very first paragraph of the decision Justice Sotomayor announced:

We conclude that the Materiality of adverse event reports cannot be reduced to a bright-line rule.[449]

The Matrixx Case Compared to Issues Raised Herein:

DIFFERENCES:
- **Consumer Choice:** In the case of Matrixx, as pharmaceutical companies, the decision to purchase and/or consume Zicam was solely at the discretion of the individual. However, in the cases presented here, neither Donna Jo, Sandra, JoAn, Susan, Shelley, Helen, nor Ben had any choice whatsoever about "consuming" their neighbors' pesticide applications. It is as Rachel Carson pointed out 50 years ago:
  We have subjected enormous numbers of people to contact with these poisons, without their consent, and often without their knowledge.[450]

- **Collusion:** In the Matrixx case there was no APPARENT government/industry collusion.
- **Third Party Product Promotion:** As noted immediately above, Matrixx and other pharmaceutical companies do not engage in the use of any third party (unless we count referring physicians) to promote their products directly to the consumer. However, in the case of the use of pesticides, the chemical companies have abundant help; namely:

---

[448] Ibid, 3.

[449] Opinion of the Court, Matrixx Initiatives, Inc, et al., Petitioners v. James Siracusano et al. On Writ of Certiorari to the United States Court of Appeals for the Ninth Circuit, 1.

[450] CF 37, Chapter 7.

1) Banking institutions requiring the use of pesticides as a condition for granting a loan to farmers for planting crops.
2) Farmer Cooperatives urging members to do likewise.

SIMILARITIES:

- **Bright-Line Rule:** While the Court rejected Matrixx's appeal to apply the bright-line rule, we have many instances of the same rule being invoked by the chemical industry and its apologists. See especially BCERF's rationale for giving pesticides the benefit of statistical doubt.[451] On the other hand note the 2001 Canadian Supreme Court ruling which rejected the bright-line rule, similar to the 2011 U.S. Supreme Court ruling in Matrixx. Note also the 2010 President's Cancer Panel Report that promotes the adoption of the Precautionary Principle, a principle that negates the bright-line rule as an operative protocol.[452]
- **Statistical Significance v. Anecdotal:** While the U.S. Supreme Court rejected Matrixx's argument that only statistically significant data is relevant, Matrixx's argument has been the rule of choice by the chemical industry, as well as USEPA. This argument has held sway in all efforts to restrict usage, as well as attempts to stablish culpability in public health litigation.

Implication # 1

Since the U.S Supreme Court and the Canadian Supreme Court have rejected the bright-line rule (and its attendant reliance on statistical significance) as the sole legal criteria in establishing culpability; and the U.S. Supreme Court has now clarified that "the source, content, and context of the reports,"[453] are to be considered relevant and material, it behooves those seeking redress to pursue with due diligence to counter chemical company bright-line arguments in courts of law, the halls of legislative bodies, the corridors of regulatory agencies, as well as the court of public of

---

[451] See Chapter 6, 7-8.
[452] See PCP 2010, 16-17.
[453] CF 453 above.

opinion. Indeed, the time is long overdue for us to take the active position advocated by Meriel Watts and the Pesticide Action Network:

> *We should not wait to obtain definitive statistical proof, because in the meantime women die unnecessarily.*[454]

Implication # 2:
The law firm SeyfarthShaw LLP concludes that:

> *Companies will now need to conduct a more holistic analysis of whether a small number of adverse events, because of their nature, would be sufficiently material to a reasonable investor to require disclosure.*[455]

Those preparing lawsuits against chemical companies or a pesticide user should develop the case for any number of adverse events which would be sufficiently material to a reasonable investor, or a reasonable legislative body, or a reasonable regulatory agency. As Adam Steinman, a law professor at Seton Hall University says. The Matrixx decision "provides plaintiffs with more ammunition...."[456]

However, as Erik J. Olson, a partner in the Morrison & Forester law firm, notes "...plaintiffs would be greatly mistaken if they came out and said that (the Matrixx decision) shows you have to consistently come out and disclose all adverse events."[457] Olson's point is well-taken and suggests the age-old rule that plaintiffs need to prepare well any and all adverse event arguments they may deem material.

---

[454] Watts, 57.

[455] SeyfarthShaw, "Matrixx: Supreme Court Rejects 'Statistical Significance' and Other Bright-Line Assessments of Materiality," March 25, 2011. www.seyfarth.com/index/cfm/fuesaction/news.pub.news.

[456] Evan Weinburger, "Matrixx Opens Door for Plaintiffs, But Only A Crack," Portfolio Media, Inc, March 22, 2011. www.law360.com/print-article/233924/section=topnews.

[457] Ibid, 3.

Implication # 3

Among the kind of data that may now have new weight are such findings as:

- The revelation that Beech-Nut Packing Company allowed detectable levels of pesticides in its baby food products.[458]
- Dr. A. Donna's 1984 study establishing a relationship between pesticides such as atrazine and ovarian cancer.[459]
- The Stokes & Brace 1988 study indicating a relationship between chemical use and cancer mortality.[460]
- All the studies mentioned at Chapter 3.
- The data at Table 1, "Synthetic Organic Contaminants: Drinking Water Standards and Health Risks or Effects."
- The data at Table 2, "Female Cancer Incidence Rate Report for Iowa (Selected Cancers: State & National Averages Compared to Fremont County)"; and Table 3, "Female Cancer Incidence & Mortality (1993-2002) (Selected Cancers and County Ranking – Fremont County)."
- The Lymphoma Foundation of America's studies noted at Chapter 6.
- The observation cited in the 2010 President's Cancer Panel Report that atrazine is the "number-one pesticide contaminant of ground water, surface water, and drinking water."[461]

Matrixx v. Siracusano has established a precedent for bringing all of the above and their like to beat in any movement to seek a limit to the growth of chemicalizing the environment and human life, as well as any effort to seek redress of damages done to individual and public health through class action law suits.

---

[458] See Chapter 1, 17.
[459] See Ibid, 26.
[460] Loc cit.
[461] See Chapter 7, 7-8, and CF 16.

Scienter & Matrixx v. Siracusano

The U.S. Supreme Court found Matrixx guilty of *Scienter;* that is, guilty of knowingly withholding relevant and material information. Part of that finding was the fact that Matrixx interfered when Dr. Bruce Jafek at the University of Colorado and his colleague planned to deliver a presentation at the American Rhinologic Society meeting in 2003. Timothy Clarot, Matrixx's vice president of research and development, had learned that Dr. Jafek and an associate were going to discuss 10 cases of patients who had taken Zicam and had experienced anosmia. Clarot sent a letter to Jafek "warning him that he did not have permission to use Matrixx's name or the names of its products."[462]

The experience of Dr. Omar Shafey, Dr. Melvin Reuber, Dennis Bishop, and Dr. Tyrone Hayes illustrate chemical company practice in bringing pressure to bear on those who "blow the whistle." The cases reported here are but a few instances of perhaps dozens where *scienter* has been manipulatively operative within the milieu of chemical company practice, i.e., bringing pressure to bear in the interest of withholding vital information. However, it is clearly more than pressure that has been employed; it is harassment accompanied with attempt at personal character assassination.

Scienter & Cipollone v. Liggett Group, Inc., 505 U.S. 504 (1992):

In the summer of 1983, New Jersey attorney, Marc Edell connected with Rose DeFrancesco Cipollone who, having been a cigarette smoker for 40 years, was dying of lung cancer. Edell ultimately persuaded the family to file a lawsuit against the three cigarette companies (Liggett, Lorillard, and Phillip Morris) whole products Rose had most commonly consumed. While many such lawsuits had would their way previously through the courts, the tobacco companies always successfully defended themselves, arguing that the plaintiffs would have had to be "deaf, dumb, and blind" to be unaware of the risks. This lawyer, however, took a completely different approach.

Edell maintained before the court that:

---

[462] Opinion, 3-4.

What mattered was not how much Rose Cipollone knew about tobacco risks; what mattered was what cigarette makers knew and how much of the cancer risk they had revealed to consumers such as Rose.[463]

For the first time in tobacco-related cancer litigation, an attorney was invoking the sciener principle. This argument won Edell the right:

To ask the courts for unprecedented access to the internal files of Phillip Morris, Liggett and Lorillard. Armed with powerful legal injunction to investigate these private files, Edell unearthed a saga of perversity. Many of the cigarette makers had not only known about the cancer risks of tobacco and the potent addictive properties of nicotine but had also actively tried to quash internal research that proved it. Document after document revealed frantic struggle within the industry to conceal risks, often leaving even its own employees feeling morally queasy."[464]

The Master Settlement Agreement (MSA) (1998) between these tobacco companies, and the 48 States who joined Rose Cipollone as plaintiffs,

Represents one of the largest liability settlements ever reached, and perhaps more profoundly, the most public admission of collusion and guilt in the history of the tobacco industry.[465]

The Matrixx pharmaceutical case and the Liggett tobacco case, while presenting themselves as models of sciener, also offer us a glimpse into one other avenue for corrective action in the interest of public health, namely that of accounting.

---

[463] Mukerjee, 270.
[464] Ibid.
[465] Mukherjee, 273; See also: http://www..ag.ca.gov/tobacco/msa.php.

The Accounting War on Truth

In their book, <u>Accounting at War: The Politics of Military Finance</u>, Warwick Funnell and Michele Chwastiak point out:

The way in which things are counted will always produce winners and losers and, therefore, accounting policies and practices are products of political struggle.[466]

In the case of Monsanto, DuPont, and Syngenta it is clearly not just a political struggle, but an economic struggle, as well. In the case of society at large, it is a public health struggle of immense proportions; and so much of it is predicated upon prejudiced accounting practices passed off as economic and scientific truths, as we have seen in the stories of scientists such as Omar Shafey, Tyrone Hayes, and Melvin Reuber, and others.

As Funnell & Chwastiak state it:

Calculative practices have frequently supplanted informed judgment to lend an appearance of objectivity to decision making. Yet, calculative practices have an inherent bias in that they only consider those aspects of a problem that can be represented quantitatively. ***One result is that issues of fairness, justice, equity and even survivability are lost.***[467]

The sad fact is that when it comes to survivability, those who are most vulnerable to becoming non-survivors of EPA and corporate decision-making regarding public safety and the wide-spread use of chemicals, are largely non-entities in the equation. As we have seen from the experience of Michelle Boone, the equations that drive EPA decisions are and have been largely set by those being "regulated."

Warwick Funnell (Professor of Accounting and Public Sector Accountability, and Head of Accounting and Finance at Kent Business School, UK) and Michele Chwastiak (Associate Professor of Accounting at the Anderson School of Management, University of

---

[466] Warwick Funnell and Michele Chwastiak, <u>Accounting at War: The Politics of Military Finance</u>, (NY & London: Routledge, Taylor & Francis, 2015), 1.
[467] Ibid, emphasis added.

New Mexico) quote Theodore M. Porter, Professor of the History of the Sciences at UCLA, in saying:

The appeal of numbers is especially compelling to bureaucratic officials who lack the mandate of a popular election or divine right. Arbitrariness and bias are the most usual grounds upon which such officials are criticized. A decision made by numbers (or explicit rules of some other sort) has at least the appearance of being fair and impersonal... Quantification is a way of making decisions without seeming to decide. Objectivity lends authority to officials who have very little of their own.[468]

Note, for example, how it was that the USAF Nuclear Targeting Guide was most likely filtered through some form of the Pentagon's "Planning, Programming, and Budgeting" (PPB) Systems Analysis process, affording little regard even to the possibility of military personnel becoming collateral damage (not to mention collateral civilian damage). As "PPB assisted with rationalizing and normalizing the arms race by converting it into a series of problems to be solved,"[469] so too with the chemical companies rationalizing and normalizing the pesticide race by converting it into a series of problems to be solved.

In the process, EPA has become somewhat of a puppet in "masking the human and social costs"[470] of the war on pests. Between the establishment of permissive Maximum Contaminant Levels (MCLs) chemical companies' persuasive role in setting EPA standards and EPA's own PPB procedures, we have a decision-making process strikingly similar to how the Pentagon and the service agencies have masked the human and social costs of war. Both the EPA and Pentagon processes are patently "free from emotions and moral judgments...."[471]

As if all this were not enough, there are all the lies and cover-ups, withholdings of truth, and the manipulation of truth, as

---

[468] Ibid, 82; quoting T.M. Porter, Trust in Numbers: The Pursuit of Objectivity in Science and Public Life, (Princeton: Princeton University Press, 1995), 8.
[469] Funnell & Chwastiak, 101.
[470] Ibid, 102.
[471] Ibid.

evidenced through, for example, the Matrixx v. Siracusano case, as well as the following example of German farmer Gottfried Glockner.

Scienter & Glockner v. Syngenta

To buttress the Matrix ruling on the principle of *scienter*, we now have the International case of Mr. Glockner in Woelfersheim, Germany, who filed a lawsuit against the Syngenta Corporation for not only withholding vital information concerning the company's genetically-modified Bt 176 corn, but also for allegedly manufacturing a "phony study."[472] Glockner lost his entire herd of 65 dairy cows due to toxicity of Syngenta's genetically-modified corn. Since filing his criminal lawsuit in 2012, Glockner seems to have lost his case, perhaps due to his previous settlement of a civil suit in 2007 with Syngenta. As of September 18, 2018, no further specific update on the case seem to be available. But, in another case with apparent scienter ramifications, law firms representing US farm workers have sued Monsanto with the accusation that the chemical giant has been "keeping silent on the chemical's (carcinogenesis) effect."[473]

A question that arises here is this: Will Farmer Glockner's case with Syngenta prove to be the Chemical Industry's "Vietnam War"? During the American participation in the Vietnam War, PPB played a defining role in decision-making regarding every dimension of US military strategy, funding, deployment, and reporting, including the infamous daily "body count" tallies. With regard to the war on pests, we have a similar but vastly different phenomenon. One might say an inverted parallel.

As it turned out in Vietnam, the body counts proved to be highly inflated, inaccurate and, as the then Secretary of Defense Robert S. McNamara admitted years later, "misleading or

---

[472] Ethan A. Huff, "Syngenta Corporation faces Criminal Charges for Covering ip Livestock Deaths from GM Corn," Nation of Change, June 27, 2012. www.nationofchange.org/syngenta-corporation-faces-criminal-charges-covering-livestock-deaths-gm-corn-1340811738.

[473] "Monsanto pushes against California listing of herbicide as cancer cause." Deutsche Welle, October 21, 2015 www.dw.com) Accessed December 6, 2015.

erroneous."[474] That was then, Now is now. Back then, the body counts were offered as evidence that the US was winning the war. Significant numbers of Viet Cong were reported as being killed every day. There was no way they could keep fighting with such devastating losses.

Today, chemical companies deny there are any deaths due to chemical toxicity. As "dead soldiers are no longer returned to the US in 'body bags' but rather (in) 'transfer tubes,'[475] those who die of pesticide-induced cancer are picked up from homes, hospitals and nursing homes by undertakers and delivered in "transfer tubes" to mortuaries and crematoria. Whereas US Vietnam military casualties' obituaries at least mentioned their deaths were due to battlefield situations, the cause of death for victims of cancer is rarely mentioned in their obituaries. And that is especially true for those whose cancer deaths may have been due to pesticides.

No matter the result of the Glockner v. Syngenta case, Gottfried Glockner and his entire herd of cows present us with a stark example of the true cost of toxicity.

The Glockner True-Cost of Toxicity

As sociologist/economist Juliet Schor puts it:

If people were paying for the ecological consequences of what they produce and consume, market decisions would be very different.[476]

In other words, if we factored in the cost of replacing Farmer Glockner's dairy herd to determine the "full cost pricing" of suing Syngenta's pesticides for the production of milk and milk-based products, we as a society might very well make alternative consumer/producer/distributor/retailer decisions. Of course, in the

---

[474] Funnell and Chwastiak, 112; quoting McNamara in Retrospect: The Tragedy and Lessons of Vietnam (NY: Vintage Books, 1996, 48).

[475] Ibid, 150; quoting T. Harper, "Pentagon Keeps Dead Out of Sight," The Toronto Star, November 4, 2003.

[476] Juliet B. Schor, Plenitude: The New Economics of True Wealth (NY: Penguin Press, 2010), 68.

case of Syngenta, any costs accrued due to court fights and legal settlement certainly would be passed on the Syngenta's customers.

Dr. Janette Sherman makes a similar point in her 1999 discussion of the apparent link between a pregnant woman's exposure to Chloropyrifos (Dursban) and children's birth defects:

> *The precautionary principle requires that when risks become known, even hypothetical risks, action must be taken to avoid exposure to those risks… Given the enormous cost of caring for affected children (running in excess of $500,000 in direct costs) the economic burdens on society are enormous: special schooling, special equipment, extensive and costly medical care, and saddest of all, loss of human potential.[477]*

Sherman's conclusions concerning the link between this particular chemical and birth defects extend beyond symptomology. She has reason to believe there is a cause-effect relationship, in that Dursban is neurotoxic and precipitates "interference with DNA and protean synthesis."[478]

Steingraber offers a model for determining the true-cost of organic vs. conventional food production:

> *In regard to cost, there is no question that organic food is considerably more expensive than conventionally produced food (in that) organic farming relies more on labor to control pests and less on chemicals… However, the higher retail price of organic food reflects the full costs of its creation, whereas the price of chemically grown food does not.[479]*

Those costs, notes Steingraber, include the costs of:
* Testing for pesticide residues,
* Removing the residues,
* Treatments for farm workers poisoned,
* Loss of honeybees and butterflies,

---

[477] J.D. Sherman, "Chlorpyrifos (Dursban) exposure and birth defects: report of 15 incidents, evaluation of 8 cases, theory of action, and medical and social aspects," Eur. J. Oncol. (Vol 4, N.6, 1999), 658.
[478] Ibid.
[479] Steingraber, # 2, 163.

* Loss of fish in rivers & streams,
* Cleaning water.[480]

Should we not add one more cost to the calculation: the enormous social and economic cost of losing productive lives due to cancer?

The Human Loss Calculus

While it is near-normal procedure for governments to calculate the cost of going to war, that is the costs of training, arming, feeding and clothing, paying, and transporting troops, governments never have calculated the costs of having gone to war in terms of estimating the cost to society of losing the productivity of hundreds, thousands, tens of thousands of lives. The EPA did settle on the estimated value of one human life as being the equivalent of $4.8 million as the agency pursued a study of the benefits and costs of the Clean Air Act.[481] It is this kind of calculus that must be exercised in determining the value of continuing the use of pesticides.

In 2011 the EPA released plans for a Second Prospective Study, noting that the Clean Air Act Amendments would by 2020 prevent:

230,000 Adult Deaths,
120,000 Emergency Room Visits
17,000,000 Lost Work Days[482]

If we assume each death prevented possesses a value of $4.8 million, as noted above, the total value of adult lives saved would come to $1 Trillion, 104 Billion; and if we assume the average

---

[480] Steingraber cites the Pimentel Study noted here for this attempt to calculate the "externalized cost" which "lead to market outcomes that are privately profitable but costly to society." (D. Pimentel, "Environmental and Economic Costs of the Application of Pesticides Primarily in the United States," Environmental Development and Sustainability 7 (2005): 229-52).

[481] Funnell & Chwastiak, 152; citing EPA, "The benefits and costs of the Clean Air Act 1990-2010" (EPA-410-R-99-001).

[482] EPA, "The Benefits and Costs of the Clean Air Act 1990-2020, The Second Prospective Study," 2011. www.epa.gov/clean-air-act-overview/benefits-and-costs... Accessed March 3, 2016.

Emergency Room Visit costs $2,168 as reported in the Atlantic Magazine,[483] the total ER costs prevented would come to $26, 040,000; and if we assume $825 as the weekly earnings of each wage and salaried workers as reported by the USW Department of Labor's Bureau of Labor Statistics[484] and divide by 5 to obtain a daily average wage ($165) and multiply that by 17,000,000 Lost Work Days, the total cost of Lost Work Days would come to $2 Billion, 805 Million; with a Grand Total savings for the United States of $1 Trillion, 132 Billion, 845 Million, 40 Thousand ($1, 132, 845, 040,000).

Now, let us consider the cancer-related death in 2015 as reported by the American Cancer Society: 1,003,859.[485] If we use the same value for each human life lost due to cancer ($4.8 million x 1, 033,859), we come to the astronomical figure of $4,818,523,200,000 ($4 Trillion 818 Billion, 523 Million, 200 Thousand); and that is for only one year's loss in human life. It is true that in no way is it contended here that all cancers are caused by pesticides. But even if we allow that perhaps only half are so caused, we still wind up with a little over a half-million people (501,930), and a monetary value of approximately $2.4 trillion lost.

For comparison purposes, let us ponder the fact that the US Department of Veteran Affairs reports the following Vietnam War mortal casualties of US Service men and women:

58,220 Vietnam War Battlefield + Other (In Theater Deaths)[486] Using the same benchmark value of $4,800,000/military personnel death as a result of our engagement in the Vietnam War, the total value of human life lost = $279 Billion, 456 Million. And that $279,456, 000,000 does not include medical costs for those who

---

[483] Lindsay Abrams, "How Much Does it Cost to Go to the ER?" The Atlantic, February 20, 2013. www.theAtlantic.com/health/archive/2013/02/how-much-does-it-cost. Accessed March 3, 20016.

[484] US Department of Labor, Bureau of Statistics, "Usual Weekly Earnings Summary," (For 4th Quarter 2015) January 22, 2016. www.bls.gov/news.release/wkyeng.nro.htm) Accessed March 3, 2016.

[485] American Cancer Society, "Cancer Facts & Figures, 2015." www.cancer.org/acs/groups/content@editorial/documents... Accessed March 3, 2016.

[486] Office of Public Affairs, US Department of Veteran Affairs, American Wars," (May 2015). www.va.gov/opa/publications/factsheets.fs_americas_wars.pdf.

were injured, nor psychological care for the thousand who have suffered from PTSD (Post Traumatic Distress Disorder).

Let us more directly compare the above three critical issues (The Clean Air Act. The Vietnam War, Cancer-related Deaths) just in terms of the number of lives SAVED or LOST and the corresponding value of human lives:

230,000 Adult Deaths Prevented by Clean Air Act
$1 trillion, 104 billion (Total Value of Human Lives SAVED)
58,220 American Vietnam War Deaths
$279 billion, 456 million (Total Value American Lives LOST)
1,003,859 Cancer-related Deaths, 2015
$4 trillion, 818 billion, 523 million, 200 thousand
(Total Value Human Lives LOST)

NOTE: With the passage of one law directed toward making the environment healthier of its citizens, the Clean Air Act, saved 171,780 more lives than were lost in Vietnam. On the other hand, combining collusion and denial, the US has avoidably suffered in one year 945,639 more deaths due to cancer than were lost during the 20 year-long Vietnam War.

Finally, a team of economists in their 2016 study entitled "Typhoid Fever, Water Quality, Human Capital Formation," conclude that an earlier 2005 study's estimates on the benefits, from governmental interventions still hold.[487] The study cited by Beech and Associates,[488] concluded that "the social return of water purification" regarding typhoid was "23-1." Beech goes on to note: "Our results indicate that the discounted increase in earnings alone (1-9%)[489] was sufficient to offset the costs of water purification."

In other words, it pays to take precautions when it comes to public health issues. And to add some other calculations: perhaps as a society, we might gain $23.00 for every $1.00 invested in

---

[487] Brian Beech, Joseph Feerie, Martin Saavedra, and Werner Troesken, "Typhoid Fever, Water Quality, Human Capital Formation," The Journal of Economic History (Vol 76, March 2016), 41-75.
[488] David Cutler and Grant Miller, "The Role of Public Health Improvements in Health Advances: The Twentieth-Century United States," Demography, No. 7, 2005, 1-22.
[489] Beech, et al, 69.

agroecology (broadly defined); and maybe another $23.00 for every $1.00 invested moving away from chemically-dependent farming and gardening. And, that could mean gaining $46 for every $2.00 just for trying to do the right thing! Just Sayin'.

The Province of Quebec, Canada: A Model for Action & Sustainability

In 2006 the Province of Quebec, by unanimous legislative consent, established what has become the Ministry of Sustainable Development, Environment and the Fight Against Climate Change.[490] While it may seem that many national, state or provincial governmental departments/ministries, once created, grow moldy and suffer bureaucratic entropy, this agency appears to fight inertia through courageous action.

David Heurtel, the then presiding Minister moved toward introducing legislation to amend Quebec's Pesticide Act, which would, among other things:

- Require all uses of atrazine to be pre-approved by an agronomist, making Quebec the first jurisdiction in North America to restrict the use of atrazine.
- Increase the existing ban of 20 pesticides from being used in urban areas to 60.
- Invoke a tax on pesticides based on levels of toxicity.[491]
- See also: "Quebec's Plan for Combatting Climate Change,"[492]

---

[490] "Quebec's Sustainable Development Act, May 2006," (Sustainable Development Act, Bill 118. www.m.gowlings.com/knowledgecentre/article.

[491] "Plan for stricter guidelines on pesticide use is welcomed by some but irks farmers," Montreal Gazette, November 22, 2015 www.montrealgazette.com/news/10cal-news/plan-for-stricter-guidelines. Accessed January 14, 2016.

[492] https://www.canada.ca/en/environment-climate-change/corporate/briefing/quebec-environment-profile.html.

The Nation of Ecuador:
A Total Holistic Approach to Sustainability

Ecuador's Constitution (2008), starting with a preamble that acknowledges the age-old roots and wisdom of all cultures, recognizes the rights of Nature, and celebrates Mother Earth (Pacha Mama) as "vital for our existence," encourages a new agricultural model based on food sovereignty and agroecology. It includes articles on the following:

- *Individuals and collectives are entitled to safe, continual access to healthful, sufficient, and nutritious foods, preferably produced locally and corresponding with their diverse cultural identities and traditions.*
- *Economic policy will have, among other goals, that of ensuring food and sovereignty.*
- *To achieve food, the Ecuadorian Government assumes responsibility for: strengthening diversification and introducing ecological and organic technologies in agricultural production.*
- *It is in the public interest and a national priority to conserve the soil, especially its fertile topsoil layer.*
- *The State will provide support to farmers and rural communities for soil conservation and restoration, as well as to develop agricultural practice protecting them and promoting food sovereignty.*
- *The public's right is recognized to live in a healthy, ecologically balanced environment that will guarantee sustainability and 'Sumak Kawsay' (living well). It is declared in the public interest to preserve the environment, conserve ecosystems, biodiversity and the security of the country's genetic heritage, prevent environmental damage and recover degraded natural spaces.*
- *All forms of appropriating collective knowledge, in the field of sciences, technologies and ancestral knowledge are prohibited. Appropriation of the genetic resources contained in biological diversity and agrobiodiversity is also prohibited.*

- *Ecuador is declared free of genetically modified crops and seeds.*
- *Public procurement will comply with criteria of efficiency, transparency, quality, environmental and social responsibility. Priority will be given for Ecuadorian products and services, particularly those from the grassroots solidarity, and from micro, small and medium production units.*
- *Additionally, the General Law of Food Sovereignty (LORSA) (amended 2010) establishes the State's obligation to promote reconversion of conventional systems into agroecological systems and encourage sustainable (agroecological) agricultural systems. It includes:*
- *Encouraging consumption of healthful, nutritious foods of agroecological, organic origin, avoiding insofar as possible the expansion of monoculture and utilization of food crops to produce biofuels, granting priority to in-country food supply. The State, and individuals and collectives, will conserve ecosystems and promote the recovery, use, conservation and development of agrobiodiversity and of the ancestral knowledge related to it.*
- *The State as well as individuals and collectives will promote and protect the use, conservation, assessment and free exchange of all native seeds.*
- *The State will also ensure applied participatory research and create an extension system, to transfer the technology generated in research, to provide technical assistance, based on dialogue and exchange of know-how with small and medium producers, valuing women's and men's knowledge.*
- *The State will promote sustainable reconversion of conventional productive processes to agroecological models and diversify production to ensure food sovereignty.*
- *The State will encourage agroecological, organic, sustainable Production, through development mechanisms, training programs, special lines of credit*

and marketing mechanisms on the domestic and external market, among others.

- *To reduce and eradicate under-nutrition and malnutrition, the State will encourage consumption of nutritious foods, preferably of agroecological and organic origin, by providing support for their marketing.*
- *The State will create the National Marketing System for Food Sovereignty and establish support mechanisms for direct negotiation between producers and consumers, provide incentives for efficiency and rationalization of marketing chains and channels. It will also work to improve conservation of food products in post-harvest and marketing processes; and will foster associative mechanisms among microentrepreneurs, microenterprises or micro, small and medium food producers, to protect them from the imposition of unfavorable conditions to market their products, regarding large marketing and industrial chains.*[493]

While Ecuador's progress in fulfilling the promises stated in its constitution is sporadic, the language itself offers a framework for a radically different approach to responsible government than anywhere else in the world. The examples of the Province of Quebec and the Nation of Ecuador are presented here as evidence that change IS possible; and that we are not necessarily condemned to the unending insanity of doing the same thing over-and-over again expecting that things will change.

---

[493] Watts & Williamson, 182-183, Box 10.1.

Afterword:

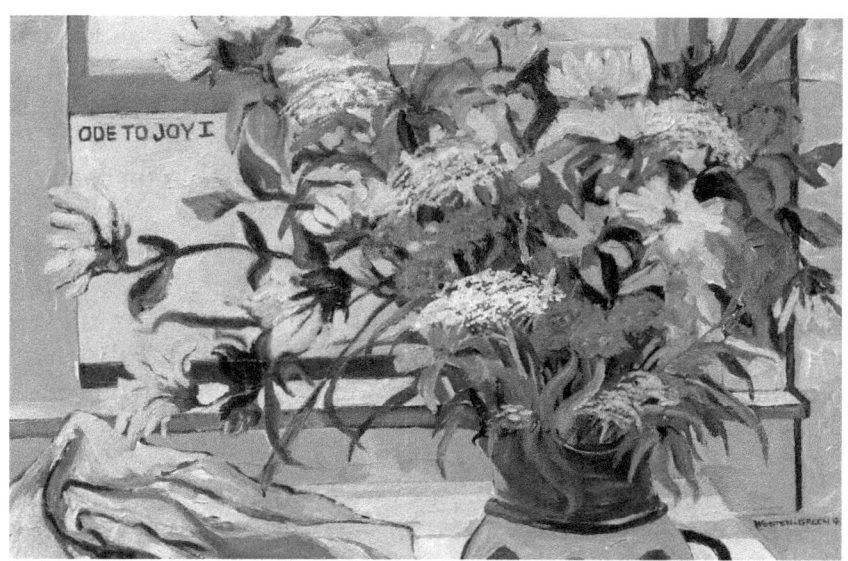

Ode to Joy
By Linda Wooten-Green

No man is an island, entire of itself; every man is a piece of the continent, a part of the main. If a clod be washed away by the sea, Europe is less, as well as if a promontory were, as well as if a manor of thy friend's or of thine own were: any man's death diminishes me, because I am involved in mankind, and therefore never send to know for whom the bell tolls; it tolls for thee.[494]
(John Donne, Meditation XVII)

Despite some appearances to the contrary, this book is not necessarily a call to take a stand for the socio-political-economic, philosophical or theological notion of "caring for creation."[495] Although, caring for all of creation is certainly a worthy call, and this author does support Pope Francis in his call for us to work for the common good. The call here is for the simple exercise of the power of common sense in avoiding avoidable death and needless human tragedy.

---

[494] http://www.online-literature.com/donne/409.
[495] Max Oelschlaeger, Caring for Creation, (Yale, 1994), 103-109.

In this same vein, it must be acknowledged that much has been said in these pages concerning cooptation and complicity with a certain recognition that THAT is the nature of politics. Politics, it has been said is the "art of the possible, the attainable…the art of the next best,"[496] the "art of making possible what is necessary,"[497] and the "repeated cooptation of the public interest by private power, especially (although not exclusively) in regard to environmental issues."[498]

Thus it is with great hope that with the suggestions rendered in Chapter 12 and the good sense of humanity we may rise a step or two above politics as the "art of the next best" and work toward the "art of the necessary," doing so with a twist on the reality that government is and always has been powered by a politics of interests. The twist is this:

When we come to realize that what we are doing to the land is, consequently, the very thing that has KILLED Grandma, Mom, Sister, Aunt, Daughter, Best Friend, Wife or Husband, then the politics of enlightened self-interest may arise like the Phoenix from the ashes of lethargy and the remoteness of political issues.[499]

Such enlightened self-interest has the potential for moving the polity from striving for some esoteric sense of the common good to a more immediate personal sense of what is necessary. As Max Oelschlaeger sees it "citizens (must) change their political behavior," but will do so ONLY when there is a public "discourse that is widely communicated, ideologically persuasive, and emotionally evocative."[500] And that is precisely where the actions taken in Malvinas, Argentina, and Haiti lead us to a glimpse of what is not just *necessary* but *possible*, especially at this moment in history, and what might be known as the dire moment of the present.

---

[496] Otto von Bismarck to Prince Meyer von Waldeck (11 August 1867) (Quotationary by Leonard Roy Frank, ed, Random House, 2011, 617.
[497] Ibid, Jacques Chirac (1995)
[498] Oelschlaeger, 57.
[499] See Oelschlaeger, 111, for a pessimistic discussion of the ability to mobilize the polity around environmental issues.
[500] Ibid, 230.

The Dire Moment of the Present

This book has been a work-in-progress since about 1998. From then until January 20, 2017, while there was much to be discouraged about in the so-called War on Cancer, there was a near-abundance of hope and promise. Let us re-cap, as it were, the discouragements, as well as the hopes and promises.

The Hopes & Promises in the War on Cancer

- *1970-US Environmental Protection Agency is created.*
- *1971-War on Cancer is declared by President Nixon.*
- *1972-US bans DDT.*
- *1974-Federal Safe Drinking Water Act becomes law.*
- *1996-US President's Cancer Panel issues first annual report.*
- *1996-Food Quality Act enacted.*

Discouragements in the War on Cancer

- *1980-Dr. Melvin Reuber fired for questioning chemical company-funded studies.*
- *1991-US exports 4+ million pounds of its own banned pesticides.*
- *1997-World Conference on Breast Cancer accuses the "Collective Cancer Establishment" of a complicity of mainstream science with government & business.*
- *1999-66% of EPA's Tolerance Reassessment Advisory Committee resign over perceived collusion between the White House, the EPA, and agribusiness.*
- *2000-Dr. Omar Shafey is fired for refusing to alter his report concerning the danger to public health from pesticide spraying.*
- *2016-Sixty-eight scientists (50 of whom have deep ties to the chemical industry, file a complaint with the European Directorate-General for Health & Food Safety charging the science behind Endocrine Disruption and the use of*

the Precautionary Principle is misguided.[501]

For example:

a. *HELMUT GREIM, Emeritus Professor of Toxicology, Technical University of Munich; and MEMBER , MONSANTO EXPERT GROUP.*

b. *COLIN BERRY, Emeritus Professor of Pathology, Queen Mary University of London; and MEMBER, MONSANTO EXPERT GROUP & CONSULTANT TO SYNGENTA.*

c. *ALAN BOOBIS, Professor of Pharmacology, Imperial College London; chaired the Joint Expert Committee of the World Health Organization and Food and Agriculture Organization <u>which provided a report</u> MINIMIZING ANY RISK OF MONSANTO'S GLYPHOSATE BEING CARCINOGENIC.*

d. *WOLFGANG DEKANT, Professor of Toxicology, University of Wurzburg; REPRESENTATIVE FOR THE FLAME RETARDANT INDUSTRY TO THE 2016 INTERNATIONAL AGENCY FOR RESEARCH ON CANCER.*

But the most discouraging and alarming of all, springs out of the current national government of the United States. There is no attempt here to provide an in-depth critique of the Administration's Environmental policies and actions. Suffice it to say, however, that the early signs indicate massive environmental and public health problems lie ahead. Simply note the headlines from the 20 months of the new Presidency & Congress concerning both actions taken and developments environmentally:

- **Republicans Are Using Big Tobacco's Secret Science Playbook to Gut Healthy Rules.** (The Intercept, February 5, 2017)
- **Donald Trump's Pick for EPA Enforcement Office Was A Lobbyist for Superfund Polluters.** (The Intercept, May 24, 2017)

---

[501] Stephane Horel, "Endocrine disruptors: Brussels' industry-linked scientists sow doubt," Environmental Health News, June 8, 2016.

- **Trump Administration to propose repealing rule giving EPA broad authority over water pollution.** (Washington Post, June 27, 2017)
- **Trump's alarming environmental rollback: what's been scraped so far.** (The Guardian, July 4, 2017).
- **Drifting crop chemical deals 'double whammy' to US farmers.** (Reuters, August 2, 2017)
- **New "Monsanto Papers' Add to Questions of Regulatory Collusion, Scientific Mischief.** (Huffington Post, August 1, 2017)
- **Gulf of Mexico Dead Zone Largest Ever, Size of New Jersey.** (KRMG, TULSA, August 4, 2017)
- **Dicamba herbicide causes problems for farmers in Kentucky: Local farmer, Jacob Goodman says Thousands of acres of crops damaged by an herbicide he didn't use.** (Paducah, WPSD-TV, August 13, 2017)
- **Millions Consumed Potentially Unsafe Water in the Last 10 Years.** (NEWS 21, August 14, 2017)
- **Collusion or Coincidence? Records Show EPA efforts to slow herbicide review came in coordination with Monsanto.** (Huffington Post, August 17, 2017)
- **Widespread crop damage from dicamba herbicide fuels controversy.** (Chemical Engineering News, August 21, 2017)
- **Pesticides linked to birth abnormalities in major study.** (The Independent, UK, August 29, 2017)
- **How Monsanto Captured the EPA (And Twisted Science) To Keep Glyphosate on the Market.** (In These Times, November 1, 2017)
- **With Kavanaugh Confirmed to the Supreme Court, Our Environment and Health Are at Risk** (National Resources Defense Council, October 6, 2018).
- **Controversy emerges over proposed bill blocking local preemption of federal pesticide regulations** (www.geneticliteracyproject.org/2018/10/09)

Yet, all the news is not bad. Again, note the headlines:

- **New claims against Monsanto in consumer lawsuit over Roundup herbicide.** (Huffington Post, June 20, 2017)

- **US state prosecutors join push to ban pesticide chlorpyrifos.** (Reuters, July 6, 2017)
- **Trump's environment and energy policies trigger storm of lawsuits.** (McClatchy Press, DC Bureau, July 12, 2017)
- **Trump's EPA Greenlit This Pesticide Linked to Brain Damage. Eight Senators Are Fighting Back.** (Mother Jones, July 26, 2017)
- **McCain's brain cancer draws renewed attention to possible Agent Orange connection.** ProPublica, Houston Chronicle, July 27, 2017)
- **Official List of 'endocrine disruptors' published.** (Connexion, France, August 2, 2017)
- **Wal-Mart puts chemicals in spotlight by joining new program.** (Bloomburg News, August 2, 2017)
- **Chemical spray damage results in record $7million negligence court payout.** (ABC Rural, August 9, 2017)
- **Greens Sue EPA over toxic chemical rules.** (The Hill, D.C., August 14, 20917)
- **How much should major polluters pay? A Case against DuPont provides a model.** (Audubon Magazine, August 16, 2017)

This book has limited ability to widely communicate its message. But there is the hope that with the stories of Donna Jo, Susan, Sandra, Shelley, Helen and Ben, and Lieutenant/Farmer Duane a certain "emotionally evocative" refrain has been added to the operatic chorus of environmental tragedy. In the end, any significant change in direction from that in which we are headed requires a fundamental change in attitude, or as the American Catholic Bishops have pleaded:

As individuals, as institutions, as a people, we need a change of heart, to preserve and protect the planet for our children and for generations to come.[502]

A Chinese Proverb , however, puts it a bit more succinctly:

If we don't change the direction we are headed, we will end up where we are going.[503]

++*+*+*+*+

Prophets vs. Profits

May we manage to avoid getting lost in semantics, as in whether we are in the midst of a cancer plague or epidemic. That is the kind of discourse which diverts attention from the fact that whatever we call it, the reality is that we do have a serious public health problem. Furthermore, we need to listen and listen well to those modern day "prophets" who are crying in the wilderness urging us to realize the urgency of the situation.

Who are those modern-day prophets? Let us make a list:
- Dennis Bishop
- Michelle Boone
- Tyrone Hayes
- Melvin Reuber
- Robert Rudd
- Omar Shafey

All speaking out in the tradition of Rachel Carson. And all of whom, have been mentioned herein at some length, detailing, in some cases, the trials they have endured for speaking out.

---

[502] U.S Catholic Conference, <u>Renewing the Earth: An Invitation to Reflection and Action on Environment in Light of Catholic Social Teaching (A Pastoral Statement, November 14, 1991)</u>. www.nccbuscc.org/sdwp/ejp/bishops.statement.

[503] Noted in Jodi Picoult, <u>Nineteen Minutes: A Novel</u> (NY: Pocket Books, Simon & Shuster, 2007), 1.

However, there are three other Whistle Blowers whose work has been mentioned often within these pages, but whose stories have not been told:

- Janette Sherman
- Sandra Steingraber
- Meriel Watts

JANETTE SHERMAN, M.D.
Retired MD, Writer, Medical Researcher, Activist, Alexandria, Virginia

Janette Sherman, MD, specializes in internal medicine and toxicology with emphasis on chemicals and nuclear radiation as Causal agents in illnesses, including cancer and birth defects. She is a graduate of Western Michigan University majoring in biology and chemistry; as well as from Wayne State University College of Michigan.

Prior to medical school, Dr. Sherman worked for the Atomic Energy Commission at UC Berkeley, and for the Navy Radiation Defense Laboratory in San Francisco. She has served on the Advisory Board for the EPA's Toxic Substances Control Act and has been an advisor to the National Cancer Institute regarding breast cancer.

Janette is the author of Life's Delicate Balance—Causes and Prevention of Breast Cancer (cited frequently in the present book) and Chemical Exposure and Disaster—Diagnostic and Investigative Techniques. She has authored nearly 75 articles in various venues.

Throughout her professional career, Dr. Sherman's credo has been that of determining the causes of illnesses and trying to prevent harm to her fellow human beings, as well as to the environment. This overriding aim of hers derives directly from the Hippocratic oath that states, among other things, *I will prevent disease whenever I can, for prevention is preferable to cure.* It is no wonder, then, that Dr. Janette Sherman is an outspoken advocate for the Precautionary Principle. She describes herself as a *Physician, Author, and Activist.* It appears this combination of credentials and passions have gotten Janette into trouble.

Her book, Life's Delicate Balance—Causes and Prevention of Breast Cancer, published in 2000 by Taylor & Francis appeared on the market under this title, rather than the one she would have preferred, a title that would have been more explicit regarding the link between cancer and pesticides. But, she lived with it. About 4 years later, Taylor & Francis decided to run a 3rd printing of the book.

Soon after the new print run, Janette received word that the publisher was pulling all copies from their inventory and would be destroying all copies. However, they did honor her request to send her the books. Taylor & Francis no longer have the book for sale. However, it is available at www.janettesherman.com.

Why the sudden change of heart by Taylor & Francis? Did it have anything to do with displeasure from heavy chemical industry financial supporters of the press? Judge for yourself.

+++++++

SANDRA STEINGRABER, Ph.D.
Ecologist, Writer, Medical Researcher, Activist
Ithaca College, Ithaca, NY

Biologist, author, activist, and cancer survivor, Sandra Steingraber writes and speaks widely about climate change, ecology, and the links between human health and the environment. Her book, Living Downstream: An Ecologist's Personal Investigation of Cancer and the Environment, published by Vintage Books/Random House in 1997, and her second edition published by Da Capo Press in 2010, are frequently cited sources in the present book. She is also the author of:

- Having Faith: An Ecologist's Journey into Motherhood, and
- Raising Elijah: Protecting Our Children in an Age of Environmental Crisis.

In Having Faith, Steingraber investigates the multiple ways in which environmental hazards pose threats to each stage of infant/child development. Through this book of hers, she calls readers to political action. The author, distinguished Scholar in Residence at Ithaca College, in fact, is a living model of one answering the call to activism. She has served time in jail after being arrested as an anti-fracking-protester and is founder of a 280-

member coalition of organizations known as New Yorkers Against Fracking. Sojourner's Magazine describes Sandra as a "poet with a knife."

Would her writing and activism have anything to do with the fact that Dr. Steingraber's second edition of <u>Living Downstream</u> was not published by the original publisher?

+++++++

MERIEL WATTS, Ph.D.
Scientist, Writer, Activist, Farmer
Auckland, New Zealand

Dr. Meriel Watts is a scientist with the Pesticide Action Network (PAN) Asia Pacific based in Penang, Malaysia (PANAP), coordinator of PAN Aotearoa New Zealand, and C0-Chair of the PAN-IPEN Pesticide Working Group. She has been busy for many years working with many NGO's on issues related to pesticides. She is a member of Australia's National Toxics Network, and is the recent recipient of the Oranga Award by the Poranga Kaupapa Trust of New Zealand "for her work in promoting positive social change without which society would be poorer."

Meriel is the author of:

- <u>Replacing Chemicals with Biology: Phasing out Highly Hazardous Pesticides with Agroecology.</u>
- <u>Poisoning Our Future: Children and Pesticides.</u>
- <u>Pesticides: Sowing Poison, Growing Hunger, Reaping Sorrow.</u>
- <u>Pesticides & Breast Cancer: A Wake Up Call.</u>

While <u>Pesticides & Breast Cancer</u> makes important contributions to this book, it was not easily obtained by this author in the United States. Dr. Watts' book was not available via Amazon.com, nor was it found via Google.com. In fact, it was not available at any American university through Interlibrary Loan. There was one copy at the U.S. Library of Congress.

Meriel was originally asked to write a brochure on what pesticides might be causing breast cancer but found there was insufficient research on the subject. After 3 years of intensive labors, her book drew together the available research, pointing the finger at

98 pesticides; that figure growing now to 99 with the subsequent identification of glyphosate as a significant promoter of the growth of breast cancer cells.

Her first book, <u>The Poisoning of New Zealand</u>, published in 1994 by Auckland Institute of Technology Press, ran into the same problem as Janette Sherman's: a chemical company threatened to withdraw funding from the Institute and soon the press was forced to shut-down. Meriel's passion for growing healthy food, free of pesticides has led her and her partner to run a small certified organic farm on Waiheke Island, providing fresh healthy food for as many locals as they can supply.

The Whistle Blowers mentioned here, it can be assumed, often feel like they are lone wolves crying in the wilderness. However, they are joined by a legion of forces including "over 1500 members of national, regional, and international science academies from 69 nations (who) signed the *World Scientists' Warning to Humanity* in 1992."[504] The Warning states:

Human beings and the natural world are on a collision course. Human activities inflict harsh and other irreversible damage on the environment and on critical resources. If not checked, many of our current practices put at serious risk the future that we wish for human society and the plant and animal kingdoms and may so alter the living world that it will be unable to sustain life in the manner that we know. Fundamental changes are urgent if we are to avoid the collision our present course will bring about.

If this book aids in some small way in averting that fatal collision, then this endeavor will be considered a success by this author.

All this having been said, this author realizes we do not inhabit an ideal world. The fact is chemicals can and do have a positive impact on society. The challenge will always be with us to affect a balance between profit and the greater good. However, as

---

[504] "Global Warming and Other Environmental Concerns," Religious Tolerance (Ontario Consultants on Religious tolerance) www.religioustolerance.org/environment.

people of all faiths and those who profess a faith in science, may we all find hope and solace in Pope Francis's

A Prayer for Our Earth:
All-powerful God, you are present in the whole universe
and in the smallest of your creatures.
You embrace with your tenderness all that exists.
Pour out upon us the power of your love, that we may protect life
and beauty.
Fill us with peace, that we may live as brothers and sisters, harming
no one.

O God of the poor, help us to rescue the abandoned and forgotten of
this earth, so precious in your eyes.
Bring healing to our lives, that we may protect the world and not
prey on it, that we may sow beauty, not pollution and destruction.
Teach us to discover the worth of each thing, to be filled with awe
and contemplation, to recognize that we are profoundly united with
every creature as we journey towards your infinite light.

We thank you for being with us each day.
Encourage us, we pray, in our struggle for justice, love and peace.[505]

And, let us be mindful, and alive with the sentiments expressed, in part, from the Buddhist Chant, the Aspiration of Shambhala:

In this time of endless gadgets, please whisper in our ear that we
descend from the clan of human decency. This world of water, trees,
rocks, sky, and earth is our heritage. This natural wonderment is our
original playground.[506]

+*+*+*+*+*+

---

[505] Pope Francis, 246.
[506] From: <u>Shambhala Chant Book</u>, Translated and Compiled by the Nalanda Translation Committee under the direction of Vidyadhara the Venerable Chogyam Trungpa Rinposhe & Sakyong Mipham Rinpoche (Halifax. Nova Scotia, Canada, 2011), 25.

APPENDIX

Table 1

Synthetic Organic Contaminants: Drinking Water Standards and Health Risks or Effects[507]

Contaminant	MCL*	Risks/Effects
• Alachlor	.002	Cancer, eye/liver damage
• Atrazine	.003	Mammary gland tumors
• Carbofuran	.04	Cancer, nervous & reproductive system effects
• Chlordane	.0002	Cancer
• Dalapon	.2	Cancer, liver, kidney damage
• 2-4 D	.07	Cancer, liver, kidney damage, skin irritations, muscle effects
• Dinoseb*	.007	Cancer, thyroid, reproductive organ damage
• Diquat*	.02	Cancer, liver, kidney, eye
• Endrin	.002	Cancer, liver, kidney, heart damage (restricted use 1980)
• Lindane	.0002	Liver, kidney, nerve, immune, circulatory damage (restricted use 1987)
• Methoxychlor	.04	Growth, liver, kidney, nerve
• Oxamylvydate	.2	Cancer, kidney damage
• Pentachlophenol	.05	Cancer, liver, kidney effects
• Picloram	.004	Cancer, kidney, liver damage
• Simazine	.07	Cancer
• Sivex 2,4,5-TP	.05	Cancer, liver, kidney damage (banned 1985)
• Toxaphene	.003	Cancer (banned 1982

---

[507] Brian A. Cohen, Tough to Swallow: How Pesticide Companies Profit from Poisoning America's Tap Water, (Environmental Working Group, 1997).
* Maximum Contaminant Levels in mg/l (milligrams/liter of water).
**"Dinoseb is a runoff of herbicides from. crop and non-crop applications."

DYING YOUNG:
A TIME-LINE & Recapitulation[508]

1938: Swiss Chemist Paul Muller introduces DDT to the world.

1940 – 1993: 4.4 billion pounds of DDT applied domestically in USA.

1940 – 1990's: Breast Cancer deaths increase 1% per year.

1941: Donna Jo is born.

1944 – 1959: Donna Jo's source of drinking water: farm & school wells.

1947: American women already running 3 times the risk of having breast cancer than was true for their great-grandmothers.

1948: Paul Muller wins Nobel Prize for development of DDT.

1949: Grape Arbor dies on Donna Jo's farm—a victim of 2-4D.

1950:   * Beech-Nut Packing Co., began allowing detectable levels of pesticide residue in baby food.
  * Syracuse University study discovers DDT feminizes roosters.

1951: DDT discovered in human breast milk.

1952: DDT used as mothproofing in dry cleaning.

1955: Sandra is born.

1955 – 1973: Sandra's source of drinking water: farm & rural school wells.

1956: Shelley is born.

1956 – 1974: Shelley's source of drinking water: contaminated community water.

1958: JoAn is born.

1958 – 1976: JoAn's source of drinking water: farm & rural schools wells.

1959: Susan is born.

  • DDT's use at U.S. domestic peak – 80 million pounds applied

1959 – 1969: Geigy Chemical Co., sales of atrazine & simazine increase from 15,890 lbs. to 64.4 million lbs. and $90 million profit in 1969.

1959 – 1977: Susan's drinking water source: farm & rural school wells.

---

[508] All that appears in this Time-Line is a re-capitulation from the preceding text.

1959 – 1988: Crops treated with pesticides increase from <20% to 96% of total.

1960 – 1980's: Herbicide use increases by 800%.

1962: Rachel Carson's <u>Silent Spring</u> warns of effects of DDT & other chemicals in the environment.

1962 – 1999: American women's breast cancer risk increases from 1 in 14 to 1 in 8.

1963: 5,150 acres of Sangre de Cristo Mountain Range sprayed with DDT.

1964: "Cancer of all types and all causes display … all the characteristics of an epidemic in slow motion … (fueled by) increasing contamination of the human environment with chemical and physical carcinogens…"

1965 – 1970: Average human intake of DDT 23 times higher than in 1982.

1970 –1994: Brain cancer, Leukemia, Hodgkin's & Non-Hodgkin's deaths highest in Midwest than for other areas in U.S.

1971: A War on Cancer is declared by President Richard M. Nixon.

1972: U.S. DDT LICENSURE LIFTED.

1973 – 1998: Childhood cancer increased by 26% for males, 37% for females.

1974:   * Federal Safe Drinking Wter Act becomes law.
   * Scientists discover chlorination by-products (CBP's) in public waters.

1974– 1998:
   *41% increase in cancer death in Fremont County, Iowa (home of Donna Jo, Sandra, Susan, JoAn & Shelley).
   *20% Iowa average increase in cancer deaths.

1976:   * 25% of American women's breast milk is too contaminated to be bottled (as a food commodity.
   *FMC Corp.begins human pesticide experiments.

1979: Rural Water Treatment facilities come to the Midwest.
   + Donna Jo is 38   + Sandra is 24   Shelley is 23
   + JoAn is 21   + Susan is 20

1979 – 2002: Small water suppliers (serving <10,000 people) exempted from CBP testing.

1980: Dr. Melvin Reuber fired from his job for questioning the findings and procedures of chemical company pesticide studies.

1984: Research links women farmers' exposure to atrazine & related herbicides to subsequent diagnoses of ovarian cancer.

1986: Maximum Contaminant Levels (MCLs) defined by EPA for most organic chemicals.

1988: Significant statistical associations found between chemical use and cancer mortality in 1497 US rural counties.

1988 – 2000: Shelley's drinking water source: farm water well.

1989: Atrazine found in 93% of Iowa water samples.

1989 – 1990: 98% of Midwest watershed streams & rivers found to have detectable levels of atrazine, metolachlor & alachlor after rainstorms.

1991: US exports 4.1 million pounds of banned pesticides, including 96 tons of DDT & 40 million pounds of endocrine disruptive chemicals.

1992: U.S. General Accounting Office estimates over 300,000 farmworkers are poisoned by pesticides annually.

1995: 	* Sampled water from faucets in Corn Belt area homes find herbicides in tap water in all but one of 29 towns & cities.

	* **Shelley is diagnosed with Cancer.**

1995 – 96: All counties in the San Luis Valley of Colorado exceed State average in late stage cancer by as much as 35%; Saguache County exceeds San Luis Valley Breast Cancer rate by 154%; Rio Grande County exceeds State average Invasive Cervical Cancer by 130%.

1996: 	* 104 Corn Belt communities with total population of 3.3 million people drank tap water contaminated with 5+ weed killers.

	* US Congress enacts Food Quality Protection Act to increase human protection from pesticide exposure.

	* **Sandra diagnosed with cancer.**

1996 – 1997: Saguache County, Colorado, exceeds State average deaths among women due to Breast Cancer by 130%.

1997: Donna Jo diagnosed with cancer.

**1998: 	* Donna Jo dies.**

	*** JoAn diagnosed with cancer.**

**2000: 	* JoAn dies.**

	*** Susan dies.**

	*** Sandra dies.**

	*** Shelley dies.**

ACKNOWLEDGEMENTS

I am overwhelmed by the courage exhibited by the patients and their families who allowed me to raise questions and issues concerning the history of the medical struggles, issue which I am sure they would much rather have avoided discussing.

Deep gratitude is extended to those who have given of their time and wisdom in reading various versions of this manuscript:

- Dr. Janette Sherman, author of <u>Life's Delicate Balance.</u>
- Dr. Meriel Watts, author of <u>Pesticides & Breast Cancer.</u>
- Dr. Werner Muller, Professor Emeritus of Science, New Mexico Highlands University, and Rancher.
- Dr. Dan Bishop, Professor Emeritus of Chemistry, Colorado State University, and Director of the International Depleted Uranium Study Team.
- Peter Anderson, editor of the Journal <u>Pilgrimage.</u>
- Vinita Hampton Wright, novelist (<u>Dwelling Places</u>), and editor at Loyola Press.
- Carol Smetana, author of <u>In Quiet Pursuit of the Good – A Profile of Alice Garrigue Masaryk.</u>
- Craig Adams, who has farmed sustainably in Wisconsin, later living out his and his wife Lucy's commitment to the cause by serving in the Peace Corps with Ecuadorian farmers.
- Martha McCabe, author of <u>Praise at Midnight,</u> and former civil rights attorney in Texas and New York.
- Rev. Dennis Hamm, S.J., Professor Emeritus of Theology, Creighton University.
- The late Dr. Curtiss Solohub, Professor, Computer Science, New Mexico Highlands University.

Finally, but by no means least, the fact that my best friend and wife, Linda's belief in this book, her constant encouragement, suggestions, and challenges have made this a better book than would have been possible otherwise. The flaws in this book are entirely of my own making.

This book would not have been possible without the cooperation of Donna Jo, Susan, Sandra, Helen, JoAn, Duane, and their families. Their honesty and no-holds barred testimony compelled this writer to widely share their stories. As noted in the Introduction, the anecdotal materials gathered from these people, put flesh on the human tragedies recounted within these pages. Oncologist and Medical Researcher, Siddhartha Mukherjee rightly states:

If the history of medicine is told through the stories of doctors, it is because their contributions stand in place of the more substantive heroism of their patients.[509]

■■

---

[509] Mukherjee, 148.

PERMISSIONS

(This author wishes to acknowledge permission to reprint the following previously published material):

- Excerpts from "Pesticide Wars – The Troubling Story of Dr. Omar Shafey," by Karen Charman (www.pmac.net/pesticide_wars); originally published at: www.tompaine.com/features/2001/11/16/index. Best accessed directly at www.karencharman.com; or, at http://mindfully.org/pesticides/fired.... Accessed February 3, 2016. (Permission granted by Karren Charman, February 15, 2016.
- "The Chemical Manufacturers Association's Environmental Illness Briefing Paper," (www.getipm.com/articles/CMA-briefing.html). Permission granted by Steve Tvedten at getpm.com.
- Excerpts from Rachel Aviv, "A Valuable Reputation: After Tyrone Hayes said that a chemical was harmful, its maker pursued him," by Rachel Aviv in The New Yorker, February 10, 2014. http://www.newyorker.com/magazine/2014/02/10/a-valuable-reputation.

All photos are photos by and of Linda Wooten-Green's paintings based on actual scenes in Fremont County, Iowa. The paintings with the split (signifying the disconnect between healthy & unhealthy farming, were part of an exhibit at the Artists Cooperative Gallery in Omaha, 2001, at the Nebraska Governor's Mansion, Lincoln, sponsored by the Nebraska Arts Council, 2002. This exhibit and others like it were held at United Methodist Church, Omaha, Immanuel Courtyard Gallery, Omaha, Knowles Mercy Retreat Center all in 2003; as well as at Hospice del Valle, Alamosa, Colorado 2005 and Vital Arts Gallery, Las Vegas, New Mexico 2006. Those paintings without the split were created later. Narratives from an early draft of this manuscript accompanied each painting.

Go to: www.lindawootengreen.com to view more photos of Linda's work.

■■

GLOSSARY

- <u>Alachlor</u>: An herbicide found in such products as Bronco, Cannon, Lariat, and Lasso. Used to control broad-leafed weeds and grasses in such crops as corn. Banned in the European Union (EU) since 2006.
- <u>Aldrin</u>: An organo-chloride insecticide used to treat soil & seed. Widely banned in 1970's.
- <u>Atrazine</u>: A triazine herbicide used to stop pre-and-post-emergence broadleaf and grassy weeds in major crops. Banned in EU and associated with drinking water contamination and birth defects.
- <u>Carbofuran</u>: a most toxic carbonate pesticide and marketed as Furadan and Curater. It is used as an insecticide for crops such as corn, potatoes, and soybeans. Banned in EU and Canada. Effectively banned in the US in 2009 due to restrictive regulatory rules.
- <u>Carbon Tetrachloride (CC14)</u>: originally used as a dry-cleaning solvent, and then used as a pesticide to kill insects in grain storage facilities. Banned in 1970 un US for use in any consumer products. Toxic to liver.
- <u>Carcinogen</u>: any substance that causes cancer.
- <u>Chlordane</u>: an organo-chlorine used as a pesticide for such crops as corn, citrus, lawns & gardens. Banned in the US in 1983 except for termite control.
- <u>Cyanizine</u>: A triazine herbicide used to control broadleaf weeds and grasses in crops such as corn and cotton. EPA has classified it as a Restricted Use Pesticide due to its presence in ground water.
- <u>Dieldrine</u>: A by-product of Aldrin. Used widely for corn, cotton, and citrus crops, as well as to control locusts, mosquitoes, and termites. Banned in US in 1987 due to harm done to humans, fish, and wildlife.
- <u>Dinoseb</u>: an organic solid used as an herbicide for post-emergence weed controls and as a corn enhancer. Associated with human reproductive problems.
- <u>Endrin</u>: an organic solid insecticide used on cotton, maize, sugarcane, etc. Used widely in US until 1980 when most uses were banned. Associated with nervous system disruption.

- Heptachlor: a residue of chlordane. Its use for crops was banned in 1978. Associated with liver damage and cancer.
- Herbicides: a substance used to kill plants and weeds.
- Insecticides: chemicals used to kill insects.
- Lindane: has been used widely as an insecticide and as a pharmaceutical for lice and scabies. Banned in 2009 by the Stockholm Convention on Persistent Organic Pollutants.
- Methoxychlor: originally intended as a replacement for DDT as an insecticide. Banned in US in 2003 and in EU in 2002. Associated with leukemia as well as endocrine disruption in children.
- Metolachlor: an herbicide effectively used for broadleaf and weed control in crops such as corn, cotton, soybeans, and peanuts. Classified by EPA as a Category C pesticide (limited evidence of its being a carcinogen).
- Pesticides: *any substance or mixture of substances intended for preventing, destroying, or controlling any pest..."* (Food and Agriculture Organization of the United Nations (FAQ) (2002).
- Rodenticides: generally known as rat poison.
- Simazine: a triazine herbicide used to control broadleaf weeds and grasses. Used for such deep-rooted crops as artichokes and asparagus. Banned in EU.
- 2,4-D: a systematic pesticide/herbicide used to control broadleaf weeds, particularly in lawns & gardens, and is the most widely used herbicide in the world. 2,4-D was a major component of Agent Orange. Dow Chemical Company presents 2,4-D as an alternative to Roundup Ready. EPA in 2007 and 2012 ruled there is no link between 2,4-D and cancer. The EU has also given it a green light. However, Sweden, Denmark, Norway, Kuwait, and the provinces of Quebec and Ontario, Canada have failed to approve its use for lawns & gardens.

INDEX TO ACRONYMS

AAP	American Academy of Pediatrics
ACSH	American Council on Science & Health
AFBF	American Farm Bureau Federation
AMA	American Medical Association
ATSDR	Agency for Toxic Substances and Disease Registry
BCERF	Breast Cancer and Environmental Risk Factors
BMP	Best Management Practices
CCL4	Carbon Tetrachloride
CDC	Center for Disease Control
CEWS	Cancer Early Warning System
CMA	Chemical Manufacturers Association
COI	Conflict of Interest
CPR	Cardio-Pulmonary Resuscitation
CREG	Cancer Risk Evaluation Guide (Cancer Risk Guide)
DCA	Dichchloroethane
DDE	Dichchloroethenelindine-a DDT breakdown product
DDT	Dichloro diphenal trichloroethane
DES	Diethylstilbestrol
EMCLG	Enforceable Maximum Contaminant Level Goal (Enforceable Limit)
EPA	Environmental Protection Agency
ESTF	Endangered Species Task Force
FAO	Food and Agriculture Organization
FDOH	Florida Department of Health
FIFRA	Federal Insecticide, Fungicide and Rodenticide Act
FQPA	Food Quality Protection Act
FWS	Fish & Wildlife Service
GIS	Geographic Information System
GJIC	Gap Junction-mediated Intercellular Communication
GMO	Genetically Modified Organism
HBMCLG	Health-Based Maximum Contaminant Level Goal (Health-Based Goal)
HHP	Highly Hazardous Pesticide
HLPE	High Level Panel of Experts on Food Security and Nutrition, UN Committee on World Food Security

IHRC	International Agency for Research on Cancer
IPM	Integrated Pest Management
ISU	Iowa State University
LFA	Lymphoma Foundation of America
LIBCSP	Long Island Breast Cancer Study Project
MCE	Multiple Chemical Exposure
MCL	Maximum Contaminant Level
MCS	Multiple Chemical Sensitivity
MSA	Master Settlement Agreement
NACA	National Agriculture Chemical Association
NAF	Northwest Area Foundation
NAMCS	National Ambulatory Medical Care Survey
NAS	National Academy of Science
NCAP	Northwest Coalition for Alternatives to Pesticides
NCFP	National Center for Food & Agricultural Policy
NCPA	National Center for Policy Analysis
NDOH	Nebraska Department of Health
NEHTS	National Environmental Health Tracking System
NHDS	National Hospital Discharge Survey
NHIS	National Health Interview Survey
NHL	Non-Hodgkins Lymphoma
NHLS	Non-Hodgkins Lymphoma Study
NOPES	Non-Occupational Pesticide Exposure Study
NRD	Natural Resource District
NRDC	Natural Resources Defense Council
NTP	National Toxicology Program
OEM	Occupational and Environmental Medicine
OPP	Office of Pesticide Programs
OSHA	Organizational Safety and Health Administration
PPB	Planning, Programming and Budgeting
PBPK	Physiologically Based Pharmacokinetics
PCP	Presidents Cancer Panel
PMAC	Pesticide Management at the Crossroads
PSR	Pesticide Sensitivity Registry
RME	Reasonable Maximum Exposure
SAP	Scientific Advisory Panel
SEER	Surveillance, Epidemiology, and End Results
SHAD	Shipboard Hazard and Defense
SLV	San Luis Valley (Colorado)
SNRD	Special Natural Resource District

SPA	Special Protection Area
SSI	Silent Spring Institute
TRAC	Tolerance Reassessment Advisory Committee
2,4-D	Dichlorophenoxyacetic acid
USAF	United States Air Force
USDA	U.S. Department of Agriculture
USGS	U.S. Geological Survey
WHO	World Health Organization
WSU	Washington State University

BIBLIOGRAPHY

A Better Row to Hoe: The Economic, Environmental, and Social Impact of Sustainable Agriculture (St. Paul, Minnesota: Northwest Area Foundation, December 1994).

Abrams, Lindsay. "How Much Does it Cost to Go to the ER," The Atlantic, February 20, 2013.

Academy of Achievement. "Rosa Parks Biography: Pioneer of Civil Rights," October 31, 2005. www.achievement.org/autodoc/page/parObio-1.

Agency for Toxic Substances and Disease Registry (ATSDR). Health Consultation: Economy Products Company Site, Shenandoah, Page County, Iowa: State of Issues and Background 1997. www.atsdr.cdc.gov/HAC/PHA/shenandoah.

_____. Public Health Assessment: Bruno Coop & Associated Properties, Bruno, Butler County, Nebraska, 1994. www.atsdr.cdc.gov/HAC/PHA/bruno.

Aiken, J. David. "Nebraska Chemigation Regulations," University of Nebraska, January 1992.

_____. "Special Ground Water Quality Protection Areas," University of Nebraska, January 1992.

American Academy of Pediatrics. "AAP Makes Recommendations to Reduce Children's Exposure to Pesticides," November 26, 2012. www.aap.org/em-us/about-the-aap/aap-press-room.

American Cancer Society. "American Cancer Society Report finds Breast Cancer Death Rate Continues to Drop," September 25, 2007. www.cancer.org/docroot/MED.

_____. "Annual Report Shows Overall Decline in U.S. cancer Incidence and Death Rates," June 5, 2001 (Atlanta, GA). www.cancer.org/docroot/MED/content?MED_2_1x_Annual_ReportShows_Overall.

_____. "Cancer Facts & Figures, 2015" www.cancer.org/acs/groups/content@editorial/documents.

American Family Physician. "Understanding Patients with Multiple Chemical Sensitivity," Letter to the Editor. www.aafp.org/990415ap/letters.

American Farm Bureau Federation. "Kleckner: EPA Must Use Sound Science for FQPA," The Voice of Agriculture, April 22, 1999. www.fb.org/news/nr/nr99/nr0422.html?print=y.

_____. "Baby Boomers are Living Proof that Pesticides are Safe," by Stuart Truelsen, The Voice of Agriculture, March 8, 1999. www.fb.org/views/focus/fo99/fo0308.html.

_____. "DDTs Place in History Being Retored," by Stuart Truelsen, The Voice of Agriculture, August 27, 2001. www.fb.org/views/focus/fo2001/fo0827.html.

American Heritage Dictionary of the English Language. (NY: Houghton Mifflin, 1979).

"Attachment 7: Collateral Damage," USAF Intelligence Targeting Guide (Air Force Pamphlet 14-210 Intelligence, 1 February 1998). www.fas.org/irp/doddir/usaf/afpam14-210/part20.

Avery, Dennis. "Why Greens Should Love Pesticides," The Wall Street Journal, August 13, 1999.

Aviv, Rachel. "A Valuable Reputation: After Tyrone Hayes said that a chemical was harmful, its maker pursued him," The New Yorker, February 10, 2014. www.newyorker.com/magazine/2014/02/10/a-valuable-reputation.

Back to the Future, MCA Home Video (1986).

Ballis, Susan S. "Did the Environment Cause My Breast Cancer?" Silent Spring Review, Summer 1999.

Bamford, James. Body of Secrets: Anatomy of the Ultra-Secret National Security Agency From the Cold War Through the Dawn of a New Century (NY: Doubleday, 2001).

Barker, Earnest (ed & trans). The Politics of Aristotle (NY: Oxford University Press, 1962).

Battaglin, William A., Earl M, Thurman, Stephen J. Kalkhoff, and Stephen D. Porter. "Herbicides and Transformation Products in Surface Waters of the Midwestern United States, Journal of the American Water Resources Association, August 2003.

BCERF. Critical Evaluation #8, April 1999. www.cfe.cornell.edu/bcerf.
_____. "Pesticides and Breast Cancer Risk, An Evaluation of DDT and DDE," Fact sheet #2, April 2001. www.cfe.cornell.edu/bcerf/FactSheet/Pesticide/fs2.ddt.cfm.

Beech, Brian, Joseph Feerie, Martin Saavedra, and Walter Troesken. "Typhoid Fever, Water Quality, Human Capital Formation," The Journal of Economic History (Vol 76, March 2016), 41-75.

Becker, Ernest. The Denial of Death (NY: The Free Press Paperbacks, 1997).

Belluz, Julia. "The way we think about cancer is outdated: Here's how to change that," Vox: Science & Health, March 2, 2016. www.vox.com/2016/3/2/11141452/living-with-cancerr-chronic.

Berry, Tomas. The Dream of the Earth, (San Francisco: Sierra Club Books, 1988).

Berry, Wendell. The Unsettling of American Culture & Agriculture (NY: Avon, 1978).

Beyond Pesticides. "Community Group Fights for Lawn Pesticide Ban," January 9, 2004.
_____. "Photo Stories," July 12, 2002. www.beyondpesticides.org/photostories/index.himl.

Beyond Pesticides Daily News Archive. "Ag Extension Agent Fired After Defending Organics," February 22, 2001. www.beyondpesticides.org/NEWS/daily_news_archive/02_201.html.

_____. "Breast Cancer and Pesticide Link," April 8, 2002. www.beyondpesticides.org/NEWS/daily_news_archive/04_08_0 2.html.

_____. "Bush Names Former Monsanto Executive as EPA Deputy Administrator," March 29, 2001. www.beyondpesticides.org/NEWS/daily_news_archive/03_29_0 1.html.

_____. "Canadian Supreme Court Rules in Favor of Residential Pesticide Ban," July 7, 2001. www.beyondpesticides.org/NEWS/daily_news_archive/07_02_0 1.html.

_____. "Former Farm Bureau Official Named to EPA," February 18, 2002. www.beyondpesticides.org/NEWS/daily_news_archive/02_1_8 02.html.

_____. "Lack of Water Quality Standards for Pesticides," March 26, 2002. www.beyondpesticides.org/NEWS/daily_news_archive/03_26_0 2.

_____. "New Book Examines True Causes of Breast Cancer," May 31, 2001. www.beyondpesticides.org/NEWS/daily_news_archive/05_31_0 1%20(2).html.

_____. "Two New Studies Reveal Dangers of Atrazine," July 2, 2002. www.beyondpesticides.org/NEWS/daily_news_archive/07_02_0 2.html.

"Bill Moyers' speech on receiving Harvard Med's Global Environment Citizen Award," Crestone Eagle, January 2005, 27.

Bird, Leonard. Folding Paper Cranes: An Atomic Memoir (Salt Lake City: University of Utah Press, 2005).

Boone, Michelle D., et. al. "Pesticide Regulation amid the influence of Industry," Bioscience (October 2014, Vol. 64, No. 10), 917-922). http://bioscience.oxfordjournals.org.

Bratton, Susan Power. Christianity, Wilderness, and Wildlife: The Original Desert Solitaire (Scranton, PA: University of Scranton `Press, 1993).

"Breast cancer study flags lawn pesticides," USA Today. Oct 21, 1999. www.usaroday.com/life/health/cancer/breast/1hcbr041.

Brody, Charlotte, et. al. "Rachel's Daughters, Searching for the Causes of Breast Cancer: A Light-Saraf-Evans Production Community Action & Resource Guide," www.wmm.com/filmCatalog/study/rachelsdaughters/pdf.

Brody, Julia Green, Joel Tickner, and Ruth Ann A. Rudel. "Community-Initiated Breast Cancer and Environmental Studies and the Precautionary Principle," Environmental Health Perspectives

The National Institute on Environmental Health Sciences, The National Institute of Health and Human Services. www.ehp.niehs.nih.gov-member.

_____. "Using GIS and historical records to reconstruct residential exposure to large-scale pesticide application," Journal of Exposure Analysis and Environmental Epidemiology (2002).

Brody, Julia G. Silent Spring Review (Winter 2002).

Brown, Valerie and Elizabeth Grossman. "Why the United States Leaves Deadly Chemicals on the Market," In These Times (November 2, 2015). www.inthesetimes.magazine.com.

"Bruno, Butler County," Center for Advanced Land Information Technologies, University of Nebraska, Lincoln. www.unl.edu/bruno.

Bruns, Mary. Sustainable Agriculture in Nebraska: A Status Report (Lyons, NE: Center for Rural Affairs, November 1986.

Canadian Network of Toxicology Centres. "Report of a Panel," Cancer 80: 1887-8, 1997. www.pmac.net/canadian.

Cancer in Colorado, 1991-1996: Incidence and Mortality by County (Colorado Central Cancer Registry, Colorado Department of Public Health & Environment, 1999).

Cancer Registry of Iowa – 1997 Cancer Report. www.public-health.uiowa.edu/shri/annual97. Also: Cancer Reports for 1998-2003

Carson, Rachel. Silent Spring (Boston: Houghton Mifflin, 1962).

"Census of Population and Housing," (www.census.gov. www.nebraska.hometown/locator.com/ne/butler/bruno.cgm.

Center for Disease Control. "EPHT: Closing America's Environmental Public Health Gap, 2007 At A Glance." www.cdc.gov/nceh/tracking/aag07.html.

_____. "World Cancer Day." www.cdc.gov/features/worldcancerday.

Charman, Karen. "Pesticide Wars – The Troubling Story of Dr. Omar Shafey." www.pmac.net/pesticide_wars. www.tompaine.com/features/2001/11/16/index. www.mindfully.org/pesticides/fired.

"Chemical Manufacturers Association's Environmental Illness Briefing Paper." www.getipm.com/articles/CMA-briefing.html.

Clement, Roland C. "Pesticides and the Living Landscape," Natural Resources Journal, October 1965, 432-34. http://lawschools.unm.edu/nrj/volumes/05/2/15_clement-pesticides.pdf.

Coalition for Alternatives to Pesticides-NL. https://pesticidealternativesnl.wordpress.com/rest-of-canada.

Cohen, Brian A., et. al. Weed Killers by the Glass: A Citizens' Tap Water Monitoring Project in 29 Cities, Environmental Working Group, 1995.

_____. Tough to Swallow: How Pesticide Companies Profit from Poisoning America's Tap Water, Environmental Working Group Group, 1997.

Cohen, Leonard. "Everybody Knows," Leonard Cohen: I'm Your Man, CBS Records (SONY), 1988.

Cohn, B.A., M.S. Wolff, P.M. Cirillo, and R.I. Sholtz, "DDT and breast cancer in young women: new date on the significance of age at exposure," Environmental Health Perspectives 2007, 115: 1406-14.

Colburn, Theo, Dianne Dumanoskin, and John Peterson Myers. Our Stolen Future: Are We Threatening Our Fertility, Intelligence, and Survival? – A Scientific Detective Story (NY: Dutton, 1996).

Colditz, G.A. "Family History, Age, and Risk of Breast Cancer: Prospective Data from the Nurses' Health Study," Journal of the American Medical Association 270, 1993, 338-43.

Collaborative on Health and Environment, "Ovarian Cancer: What We Know," 2004. www.protectingourhealth.org/newacience/ovariancancer/ovarian

Connarroe, Joel, ed. Six American Poets (NY: Random House, 1991).

Cook, Alan R. and Peter D. Dresser, eds. Cancer Sourcebook for Women (Detroit: Omnigraphics, Inc., 1996).

Cutler, Cutler, and Miller, "The Role of Public Health Improvements in Health Advances: The Twentieth Century United States," Demography, No. 7, 2005, 1-22.

Daniels, Dr. Catherine. "Pesticide Sensitive Registry in Washington and Other States". www.tricity.wsu.edu/aenews/Mar99AENews.

Davies, J.E. and R. Doon. "Human Health Effects of Pesticides," in Silent Spring Revisited.

Department of Economics, Iowa State University. "Census of Agriculture – Fremont County," Iowa Peofiles: Public Resources Online (Ames: ISU). www.profiles.iastate.edu/data/census/county/agcensus.asp?sCounty=19071.

"Depleted Uranium Bill Introduced into Congress," The Lone Star Iconoclast Online www.iconoclast-texas.com/news/22nov04.

Donna, Dr. A., et. al. "Ovarian Mesothelial Tumors and Herbicides: A Case-Control Study," Carcinogenesis 5 (1984).

_____. "Triazine Herbicides and Ovarian Epithelial Neoplasms," Scandinavian Journal of Work Environments and Health 15 (1989), 47-53.

Douglas, James W. JFK and the UNSPEAKABLE: Why He died and Why It Matters (Maryknoll, NY: Orbis Books, 2008).

Duhigg, Charles. "Millions in U.S. Drink Dirty Water, Records show," NY Times, December 8, 2009.

Earth & Sky (November 27, 2001), (authored by Eleanor Imster, Narrated by Joel Bloch & Debra Bird). www.earthsky.com/Shows. Via FM Radio, KVNO, Omaha, NE.

_____. "More Information on the 'Dead Zone.'" www.earthsky.com/2001/esmi011127.

Earthjustice. "Columbian Court Orders Suspension of Coca Spraying," June 26, 2003. www.earthjustice.org/news/print.html?ID=620.

Eisenberg, Evan. The Ecology of Eden (NY: Alfred Knopf, 1998).

Ember, L. "Pollution Prevention: Study Says Chemical Industry Lags," Chemical and Engineering News (20 March 1995).

Endocrine Disruptor News Archive: January-June 1999. www.som.tulane.edu/ecme.eehome/Archive.

"Enola Gay Chronology," at "Enola Gay/The Plane," www.theenolagay.cim/plane.

Environmental Working Group. "EPA Sued for Illegally Taking Direction From Chemical Industry Group." www.earthjustice.org/news/documents/1-04/FIFRA.complaint.pdf%20.

_____. "Protecting Farm Workers From Pesticides," 2004. www.earthjustice.org/campaign/print.html?ID=9.

Environmental Working Group and U.S. Public Interest Research Group. "Consider the Source: Farm Runoff, Chlorination Byproducts and Human Health," October 2001.

_____. "A national assessment of tap water quality," September 18, 2009. www.ewg.org/tap_water/findings.php.

Epstein, Samuel S. Cancer-Gate: How to Win the Losing Cancer War (Amityville, NY: Baywood Publishing Company, 2005).

_____. Politics of Cancer Revisited (East Ridge Press, 1998).

Exposure: Environmental Links to Breast Cancer. Available through Women's Healthy Environments Network (WHEN). http://www.womenshealthyenvironments.ca/films.

Fagan,, Dan, Marianne Lavalle, and the Center for Public Integrity. Toxic Deception: How the Chemical Industry Manipulates Science, Bends the Law, and Endangers Your Health, (Secaucus, NJ: Carol Publishing Group, 1996).

Foster, John Bellamy, and Brett Clark. "Rachel Carson's Ecological Critique," Monthly Review (February 2008, Volume 59, Issue 09). http://monthlyreview.org/2008/02/01/rachel-carsons-ecological-critique.

Frayssinet, Fabianna. "Argentine Activists Win First Round Against Monsanto." Inter Press News, January 2014. www.ipsnews.net/2014/01/argentine-activists-win-first-round-monsanto-plant/

Freunkel, Susan. "Pesticides and the Young Brain," The Nation (March 31, 2014, 12-22.

Funnell, Warwick and Michelle Chwastiak. <u>Accounting at War: The Politics of Military Finance</u> (NY & London: Taylor & Francis, 2015).

Galeano, Eduardo. <u>Children of the Days: A Calendar of Human History</u> (NY: Nation Books, 2013.)

Gallagher, Erin. "Malvinas, Argentina: 200 Day Blockade Against Monsanto," Revolution News, April 5, 2014. http://revolution-news.com?malvinas-argentina-200-day-blockade-monsanto.

Geiser, K. "The Greening Industry: Making the Transition to a Sustainable Economy," <u>Technology Review,</u> August-September 1991, 65-72.

"Genetics," www.breastcancer.org/risk/factors/genetics. Sept. 17, 2012.

Geyer, Alan and Barbara Green. <u>Lines in the Sand: Justice and the Gulf War</u> (Louisville, KY: Westminster/John Knox Press, 1992.

Georgiadis, Pavlov. "Monsanto on trial for crimes against nature and humanity," The Ecologist, December 6, 2015. www.theecologist.org/News/news_round_up/298657/Monsanto_on_trial.

Geyer, Alan and Barbara Green. <u>Lines in the Sand: Justice and the Gulf War</u> (Louisville, KY: Westminster/John Knox Press, 1992.

"Global Warming and Other Environmental Concerns," Religious Tolerance (Ontario Consultants on Religious Tolerance) www.religioustolerance.org/environment.

Goffman, John W. and Egan O'Connor. "Cancer in the Family: Does Each Case Require More Than One Cause? The Likelihood of Co-Action," Committee for Nuclear Responsibility, Inc. www.ratical.org/radiation/CNR/CoAction.html.

Goldman, Lynn R. "Geographic Analysis: Cancer Mortality Maps, U.S., 1970-1994.

GoPetition: Changing the World: Agent Orange—Vietnam Memorial Wall." www.gopetition.co.uk/petitions/agent-orange-vietnam-wall-memorial.html.

Goudy, Willis, Sandra Chawat Burke and Margaret Hansen. <u>Iowa's Counties: Selected Population Trends, Vital Statistics and Socioeconomic Data</u> (Census Service, Department of Sociology, Iowa State University, October 2000), 122-125.

Gould, Pamela. "Ex-agent, Tech settle suit: School agrees to pay Bishop $13,767," Fredericksburg Free Lance-Star, June 5, 2001. www.fredericksburg.com/NEWS/FLS/2001/06200/06052001/302083.

Great Lakes Commission des Grands Lacs www.glc.org/about.

Grossman, Elizabeth. "Why the EPA Pulled a New Pesticide for GMO Corn and Soy," Civil Eats, December 1, 2015. www.civileats.com/2015/12/1/why-the-epa-pulled.

Grudin, Robert. The Grace of Great Things – Creativity and Innovation (NY: Ticknor and Fields, 1990).

Hacker, Jacob S. and Paul Pierson. Winner-Take-All Politics: How Washington Made the Rich Richer – And Turned its Back on the Middle Class (NY: Simon & Schuster, 2010).

Harper, T. "Pentagon Keeps Dead Out of Sight," The Toronto Star, November 4, 2003.

Hartmann, Thomas. What Would Jefferson Do?: A Return to Democracy (Nevada City, CA: Harmony Books, 2004).

Hiles, Marv. The Way Through: Contemplative Companion #14 Late Autumn, 2003.

Horel, Stephane. "Endocrine disruptors: Brussels' Industry-linked scientists sow doubt," Environmental Health News, June 8, 2 2016.

Hueper, W.C., and W.D. Conway. Chemical Carcinogenesis and Cancers (Springfield, IL: Charles Thomas, 1964).

Huff, Ethan A. "Syngenta Corporation faces Criminal Charges for Covering up Livestock Deaths from GM Corn," Nation of Change, June 27, 2012. www.nationofchange.org/syngenta-corporation-faces-charges-covering-livestock-deaths-gm-corn-1340811738.

"Human Development: Abundance and Scarcity – A Pastoral Letter on the Economy of Northeast Nebraska," by Archbishop Daniel Sheehan, Archdiocese of Omaha, January 11, 1991.

Human Pesticide Experiment, June 2005 (United State House of Representatives, Committee on Government Reform – Minority Report, Special Investigations Division, United States Senate, Office of Senator Barbara Boxer, Environmental Staff). www.Democrats.Reform.House.Gov. www.Boxer.Senate.Gov.

Insider, The. Walt Disney Video, 2000.

Integrity of Science Database www.cspinet.org.

"Intercellular Communication and Prostate Carcinogenesis," American Society of Clinical Oncology. www.sco.org/portal/site/ASCOv2/template.RAW/menuitem.a1c60e3.

Iowa Association of Naturalists. Iowa Agricultural Practices & the Environment,(Iowa Environmental Issues Series), September 1998.

_____. Iowa Water Pollution (September 1998).

Iowa Department of Natural Resources, Geological Survey Bureau. "The Iowa State-Wide rural Well-Water Survey: Water-Quality Data:

Initial Analysis (Abstract)," September 19, 1990.
www.igsb.uiowa.edu/gsbpubs/abstracts/TIS-19.

Ivory, Danielle. "EPA Fails to Inform Public About Weed-Killer in Drinking Water," Huffington Post, August 23, 2009. www.huffingtonpost.com/2009/08/23/epa-fails-to-inform-publi_n_26686.

Jackson, Wes. "Farming In Nature's Image: Natural Systems Agriculture," in The Fatal Harvest Reader.

Kahn, Si. And Elizabeth Minnich. The Fox in the Henhouse: How Privatization Threatens Democracy. (Redmond, WA: Berrett-Koehler Publishers, 2005).

Kepner, John. "Around the Country – Pesticides and You" (Vol 22, N0.3, 2003) (Beyond Pesticides).

Kimbrel, Andrew. "Organic and Beyond," Bioneers Letter, Autumn 2003.

Klein, Naomi. This Changes Everything: Capitalism vs. The Climate (NY: Simon & Schuster, 2014).

Krantz, Laura. "Harvard professor failed to disclose connection," Boston Globe, October 1, 2015. www.bostonglobe.com/metro/2015/10/01/harvard-professor-failed-disclose-monsanto-connection.

Kristof, Nicholas D. "New Alarm Bells About Chemicals and Cancer," The New York Times, May 6, 2010.

_____. "The Cancer Lobby: WHO knew that carcinogens had their own lobby in Washington?" The New York Times, October 6, 2012. www.nytimes.com/2012/10/07/opinion/Sunday/kristof-the-cancer-lobby.

Kroese, Ron. "Industrial Agriculture's War Against Nature," in The Fatal Harvest Reader.

Kubler-Ross, Elizabeth. On Death and Dying (NY: Macmillan, 1969).

Lanphear, Bruce. "Little things matter: the impact of toxins on the developing brain," www.youtube.com/Watch?v=E6KomAb2/BW.

_____. "Pesticides at even low levels harmful to children," The Hindu Times, September 7, 2015. www.thehindu.com/news/national/kerala/pesticides-at-even-low-levels-impact-children.

Laug, E.P., et. al. "Occurrence of DDT in Human Fat and Milk," A.M.A. Archive of Industrial Hygiene and Occupational Medicine 3(1951).

"Legal Action by Vietnamese Agent Orange Victims Inevitable," World AFP, February 8, 2003. www.panna.org.

Lerner, Sharon. "EPA used Monsanto's Research to Give Roundup A Pass," The Intercept, November 3, 2015. http://theintercept.com/2015/11/03/epa-used-Monsanto-funded-research.

Lexchin, J., et. al. "Pharmaceutical industry sponsorship and research outcome and quality: Systematic Review," BMJ 326: 1167-1170.

Lichtenstein, P., et. al. "Environmental and heritable factors in the causation of cancer – analyses of cohorts of twins in Sweden, Denmark, and England," New England Journal of Medicine, 2000. 343(2); 78-85.

Lipman, Larry and Jeff Nesmith. "Anthrax strategy assailed on Hill," Atlanta Journal Constitution, October 24, 2001.

Lipton, Bruce. The Biology of Belief: Unleashing the Power of Consciousness, Matter, and Miracles (Santa Rosa, CA: Hay House, 2005).

Luoma, Jon. "Under the Influence: Is Industry becoming an inside player at the world's leading research center on carcinogens?" NRDC, On Earth, Fall 2002. www.nrdc.org/onearth/02fal/iarc.asp.

Lymphoma Foundation of America. "Do Pesticides Cause Lymphoma?" 2001. www.lymphomaresearch.org.

Lynch, Henry T. and Jane. "Lynch Syndrome: Genetics, Natural History, Genetic Counseling, and Prevention," Journal of Clinical Oncology (Vol. 18, Issue 9, November 2000, 19-31. www.jco.org/cgi/content/abstract/18/suppl_1/19s.

Mara, G. and C.R. Boland. "Hereditary Nonpolyposis Colorectal Cancer: The Symptoms, the Genes, and Historical Perspectives," Journal of the National Cancer Institute 87 (1995), 1114-1125.

Marco, Gino G. ed. Silent Spring Revisited (Washington, DC: American Chemical Society, 1987).

Martin, Andrea. "Reclaiming Our Birthright," Silent Spring Review, Fall 2000.

Martin, Brian. "Critics of pesticides: whistle blowing or suppression of dissent?" Philosophy and Social Action,(Vol. 22, No. 3, July-September 1996. www.uow.edu.au/arts/sts/bmartin/pubs/96psa.html.

Marty, Diane. "Getting On Our Nerves: Researchers Find a Connection Between Parkinson's Disease and Pesticides." www.emagazine.com/january-february/2002/0102g/health.html.

Matrixx Initiatives, Inc., et. al., v. Siracusano, et. al. Certiorari to the United States Court of Appeals for the Ninth Circuit. No.09-1156. Argued January 10, 2011 – Decided March 22, 2011. www.supremecourt.gov.

McCampbell, Ann. "Multiple Chemical Sensitivities Under Siege," www.getipm.com/personal/mcs-campbell.

McGheehin, Michael A., Judith Qualters and Amanda Sue Nakar. "National Environmental Public Health Tracking Program: Bridging the Information Gap," Environmental Health Perspectives, (Volume 112, Number 14, October 2004), 1409-1413. www.ehp.niehs.nih.gov/members/2004/71409/7114.

McNamara, R.S. In Retrospect: The Tragedy and Lessons of Vietnam (NY: Vintage Books, 1996)

Metcalfe, Les. "Flexible Federalism," a paper presented at the Conference on Civil Service Systems in Comparative Perspective," Indiana University, Bloomington, Indiana 5-8 April 1997 (CSSCP, Conference #403-97). www.indiana.edu/~cstc/metcalf1.

Mohan, Megha. "Cancer Cases: Pesticides the Culprit," Hindustan Times, September 7, 2004.

"Monsanto: Internationals Monsanto Tribunal in the Hague, October 16, 2015," www.Monsanto-tribunal.org.

"Monsanto pushes against California listing of herbicide as cancer cause," Deutsche Welle, October 21, 2015. www.dw.com.

Montague, Peter. "Living Upstream – a review," Rachel's Environment & Health Weekly, #565, September 25, 1997. www.pmac.net/downstream.

Montgomery County, Maryland. "Special Protection Areas." www.montgomeryclountymd.gov/deptmpl.

Moss, Ralph. "Our Futile War on Cancer," New Scientist (December 16, 2006). www.newscientist.com/channel/health/mg19225825.400-our-futile-war-on-cancer.

Moyers, Bill. Speech on Receiving Harvard Meds Global Environment Citizen Award, Crestone Eagle, January 2005.

Mukherjee, Siddhartha. The Emperor of All Maladies: A Biography of Cancer (NY: Scribner, 2010).

Museum of the Cherokee Indian, Cherokee, North Carolina. www.cherokeemuseum.org.

"NAFTA pesticide ban challenge settled without money," CBC News Montreal (May 30, 2011). www.cbc.ca/news/canada/montreal/nafta-pewsticide-ban-challenge-without-money-1.1005002.

National Cancer Institute. "State Cancer Profiles." www.statecancerprofiles.cancer.gov/incidencerates.

_____. "Understanding Gene Testing," National Health Institute Pub. 96-3905 (Bethesda, MD: National Cancer Institute, 1995).

National Center for Policy Analysis. "Misconceptions About Environmental Pollution, Pesticides and the Causes of Cancer," (NCPA Report No. 214). www.ncpa.org/studies/s214.

_____. "About the NCPA," www.ncpa.org/abo.

National Conference of Catholic Bishops. Renewing the Earth: An Invitation to Reflection and Action on Environment in Light of Catholic Social Teaching – A Pastoral Statement5 of the United States Catholic Conference, (November 14, 1991.)

National Pesticide Retrieval System. www.ppis.ceris.purdue.edu/npublic.

National Pollution Prevention and Toxics Advisory Committee, Broader Issues Working Group. Initial thought starter: How can EPA more efficiently identify potential risks and facilitate risk reduction decisions for non-HPV chemicals? (October 6, 2005). www.epa.gov/oppt/npptac/pubs/finaldraftnonhpvpaper051006.PDF.

National Toxicology Program Report on Carcinogens. (11th ed.) Research Triangle Park (NC): National Institute for Environmental Health Sciences, 2005. http://ntp.niehs.nih.gov.

"New Study Links Monsanto's Roundup to Cancer," (June 1999). www.biotech-info.net/glyphosate_cancer.

Noriega: God's Favorite(Showtime/Third Row Center films, 2000).

North Carolina Cooperative Extension Service. "NWQEP Notes: The NCSU Water Quality Group Newsletter (July 1993, #60). www.bae.ncsu.edu/programs/extension/wqg/issues/60.

Northwest Area Foundation www.nwaf.org/About.

Nuland, Sherwin. How We Die: Reflections on Life's Final Chapter (NY: Alfred Knopf, 1994; Vintage, 1995).

Nussbaum, Paul. "New Orleans' growing danger: Wetlands loss leaves city a hurricane away from disaster," Philadelphia Inquirer, October 8, 2004. www.hurricane.lsu.edu/_in_the_news/phillyinquirer100804.

O'Brien, Irene. "Bruno, Butler County." www.casde.unl.edu/history/counties/butler/bruno.

Oelschlanger, Max. Caring for Creation (New Haven: Yale University Press, 1994).

Office of Pesticide Programs, Environmental Protection Agency. "The Triazine Pesticides: Atrazine, Cyanazine, Simazine, and Propazine," (August 1999). www.epa.gov/pesticides/citizens/triazine.

_____. "Acetochlor: Desk Statement," (March 11, 1994). www.epa.gov/oppefed1/acero/index.

Office of Public Affairs, US Department of Veteran Affair. "Amerian Wars," (May 2015). www.va.gov/opa/publications/factsheets_fs_americas_wars.pdf.

Pazniokas, Mark and Dennis Williams. "Navy admits what crews knew: Tests Biological," Atlanta Journal Constitution, October 21, 2001.

'Pesticide Sensitivity Registries: Descriptive Summary of a Survey of State Pesticide Sensitivity Registries and Evaluation of Louisiana's Registry for Pesticide Hypersensitive Individuals," Louisiana Department of Health and Hospitals, Office of Public Health, Section of Environmental Epidemiology and Toxicology, December 2003. www.dhh.Louisiana.gov/offices/publications/pubs-05/FINALHypersensitivityRegistry.

"Pesticide Tests on Humans banned," Omaha World Herald (December 16, 2001.

"Photo Stories," July 12, 2002. www.beyondpesticides.org/photostories/index. see also: https://www.dailytelegraph.com.au/news/nsw/landmark-legal-case-will-probe-the-link-between-parkinsons-disease-and-insecticide-sprays-used-on-longhaul-flights/news-story/8bed79471fc461cfaf1680ebc82265cf.

Picoult, Jodi. Nineteen Minutes: A Novel (Pocket Books, Simon & Schuster, 2007.

Pimentel, D. "Environmental and Economic Costs of the Application of Pesticides Primarily in the United States," Environmental Development and Sustainability7 (2005): 229-252.

"Plan for stricter guidelines on pesticide use is welcomed by some but irks farmers," Montreal Gazette, November 22, 2015. www.montrealgazette.com/news/10cal-news/plan-for-stricter-guidelines.

Pollan, Michael. The Botany of Desire: A Plant's-Eye View of the World (NY: Random House, 2001).
_____. The Omnivore's Dilemma: A Natural History of four Meals (NY: Penguin Press, 2006).

Pope Francis. Laudato Si: On Care for Our Common Home (Vatican Press, May 24, 2015).

Porter, T.M. Trust in Numbers: The Pursuit of Objectivity in Science and Public Life (Princeton, NJ: Princeton University Press, 1995).

President's Cancer Panel. Environmental Cancer Risk: What We Can Do Now(2008-2009 Annual Report, (U.S. Department of Health and Hyman Services, National Institute of Health, National Cancer Institute, April 2010.

"Public Health Assessment: Bruno Coop & Associated Properties, Bruno, Butler County, Nebraska." www.atsdr.cdc.gov/HAC/PHA/bruno.

"Quebec's Sustainable Development Act, May 2006."
www.m.gowlings.com/knowledgcentre/article.
Quigley, Winthrop. "The Word 'War' is a rhetorical minefield,"
Albuquerque Journal, December 10, 2015, 1,3.
Quotationary, Leonard Roy, ed (NY: Random House, 2001).

Rachel Carson. (A PBS, An American Experience Production, 2017, 113m.
Regenstein, Lewis G. Cleaning Up America (NY: Acropolis Books,
1993).
"Rio Declaration on the Environment and Development, Principle
15.137," 14 June 1992. www.iisd.org/rio+5/agnda/declaration.
Riordan, T.O. and J. Cameron (eds.). Interpreting the Precautionary
Principle (London: Earthscan, 1994).
Rudd & Genelly. "Pesticides: Their Use and Toxicity in Relation to
Wildlife," (California Department of Fish & Game, !956).
Rudd, Robert L. Pesticides and the Living Landscape (Madison: The
University of Wisconsin Press, 1964).
Ruffle, Ricarda. "Digging for Alternatives: An Analysis of Potato Pest
Management Research at Two Northwest Land Grant
Universities," (Northwest Coalition for Alternatives to
Pesticides) www.pesticide.org/DiggingFor Alteerrnatives.pdf.

Safe Chemicals Act 2013. www.govtrack.us/congress/bills/113/s696/text.
Salter, Jim. "Report: Army tested chemicals on St. Louis in 1950's,"
October 4, 2012. www.knoxnews.com/news/2012/octt/04/report-
army-tested-chemicals.
Schlanger, Zoe. "Does the EPA Favor Industry When Assessing
Chemical Dangers?" Newsweek, September 3, 2014.
http://www.newsweek.com/does-epa-favor-industry-when-
assessing-chemical.
Schor, Juliet B. Plenitude: The New Economics of True Wealth (NY:
Penguin Press, 2010).
Seeger, Pete. "The Columbia Concert, 1961," Pete Seeger: In His Own
Words, Selected and Edited by Rob & Sam Resenthal (Boulder,
CO: Paradigm Publishers, 2012), 251.
SEER Manual. www.public-health.uiowa.edu/shri/MAN33-55.
SeyfarthShaw, "Matrixx: Supreme Court Rejects 'Statistical significance'
and Other Bright-Line Assessments of Materiality," March 25,
2011." www.seyfarth.com/index.cfm/fuse.action/news.pub.news.
Sherman, Janette D. Life's Delicate Balance: Causes and Prevention of
Breast Cancer (NY: Taylor & Francis, 2000).
Sherman, JD. "Chlorpyrifos (Dursban) exposure and birth defects: Report
of 15 incidents, evaluation of 8 cases, theory of action, and
medical and social aspects," Eur. J. Oncol (vol. 4, N.6, 1999)
658.
Silent Spring Institute. "New Computer Tools Assesses Women's
Pesticide Exposures," February 27, 2002.

Simmons, Brigadier General James. <u>Saturday Evening Post</u>, January 6, 1945 in <u>The Fatal Harvest Reader.</u>

"Socio-environmental conflicts: Monsanto in Malvinas, a badge," April 23, 2017. http://www.laoz.com/ar/loultimo.

Sorg, Barbara A. "Multiple Chemical Sensitivities," <u>Agrichemical and Environmental News,</u> March 1999, Issue N.155 (Cooperative Extension, Washington State University. www.tricity.wsu.edu/aenews/Mar99AENews; www.aenews.wsu.edu.

Souder, William. <u>On a Farther Shore: The Life and Legacy of Rachel Carson</u> (NY: Crown Publishers, 2012.)

Spade, Linda. "GMO's in the SLV," Crestone Eagle, January 2005.

<u>State Farm Road Atlas</u> (1997 Rand McNally).

Steingraber, Sandra. <u>Living Downstream: An Ecologist's Personal Investigation of Cancer and the Environment</u> (Philadelphia: De Capo Press, 2010).
_____. <u>Living Downstream: An Ecologist's Personal Investigation of Cancer and the Environment</u> (NY: Vintage Books, 1998).

Stokes, C.S. and K.D. Brace. "Agricultural Chemical Use and Cancer Mortality in Selected Rural Counties in the USA," <u>Journal of Rural Studies 4</u> (1998): 239-47.

Strange, Marty. <u>Family Farming: A New Economic Vision</u> (Lincoln: University of Nebraska Press, 1988).

Syrenglas, Chris. "Lawn Pesticides," Interdisciplinary Minor in Global Sustainability, Senior Seminar (Univesity of California, Irvine, 1997). www.mamba.bio.uci.edu/~pjbryant/global/sen_sem/syren97.

<u>Universal Almanac 1996, The.</u>

University of Iowa. "The 2005 Iowa Fact Book." www.public.iowa/Factbook/2005/CANCER.PDF.

"Upper Elkhorn Natural Resources District, The." www.uenrd.org.

Urbina, Ian. "Panel Suggests Using Inmates in Drug Trial," NY Times, April 13, 2006.
_____. "Think Those chemicals Have Been Tested?" NY Times, April 13, 2013. www.nytimes.com/2013/04/14/Sunday-review/think-those-chemicals-have-been-tested.

USA Today. www.usatoday.com/life/health/cancer/breast/hcbr041.

"USAF Intelligence Targeting Guide," AF Pamphlet 14-210, February 1, 1998.

U.S. Catholic Conference. <u>Renewing the earth: An Invitation to Reflection and Action on Environment in Light of Catholic Social Teaching (A Pastoral Statement, November 14, 1991.</u> www.nccbuscc.org/sdwp/ejp/bishops.statement.

US Department of Labor, Bureau of Labor Statistics. "Usual Weekly Earnings Summary," (For 4th Quarter 2015) January 22, 2016. www.bls.gov/news.release/wkyeng.nr0.html.

"Use of Pesticides in New Mexico." www.farmworkers.org/pestieng.

U.S. Environmental Protection Agency. "Selected Findings and Current Perspectives on Urban and Agricultural Water Quality by the National Water-Quality Assessment Program," April 2001 (FS-047-01.)

_____. "Environmental Policy and Technology." www.epa.gov/oppfead1/trac.

_____. "Federal Insecticide and Rodenticide Act, 2008.

_____. "Surf Your Watershed." www.cfpub.epa.gov/surf/locatee/streamsperhuc_search.

_____. "The Benefits and Costs of the Clean Air Act 1990-2010," (EPA-410 R-99-001.

_____. "The Benefits and Costs of the Clean Air Act 1990-2020, The Second Prospective Study," 2011. www.epa.gov/clean-air-act-overview/benefits-and-costs.

USGS Survey, 1999, "The Quality of Our Nation's Waters – Nutrients and Pesticides," (USGS Circular 1225).

USGS. "Water Quality in the Central Nebraska Basins, Nebraska, 1992-95. www.water.usgs.gov/pubs/circ1163

US Veteran Dispatch (www.usvetdsp.com); Veteran's Book and Video Store, www.lewispublishing.com.

Van Andel Research Institute (2009, August 14). "Cancer Mortality Rates Experience Steady Decline: Conventional Method May Underreport Declining Death Rate for All Age Groups. Science Daily. www.sciencedaily.com/releases/2009/08/090813142359.html.

Wargo, John. Our Children's Toxic Legacy: How Science & Law Fail to Protect us from Pesticides (New Haven: Yale University Press, 1996).

Warren, Michael and Natacha Pisarenko. "Argentines link health problems to agrochemicals," www.kob.com/article/stories/S3197070.

Water Quality Control Division, Colorado Department of Health and Environment. "Water Quality in Colorado, 2000."

Watts, Meriel and Stephanie Williamson. "Replacing Chemicals with Biology: Phasing out highly hazardous pesticides with agro ecology," (Pesticide Action Network International, Penang, Malaysia, 2015) [Published by PAN Asia and the Pacific –PAN AP] on behalf of PAN International.

Watts, Meriel. Pesticides & Breast Cancer: A Wake Up Call (Penang, Malasia: Pesticide Action Network [PAN Asia & the Pacific], 2007), 9.

Weinberger, Evan. "Matrixx Opens Door for Plaintiff, But Only A Crack," Portfolio Media, Inc. March 22, 2011. www.law360.com/print-articl/23324?section=topnews.

"Who was Nicole Bruinsma? Why is this Story So Important?" www.precautionaryprinciplefkilm.com/project-in-depth.

Wildavsky, Aaron B. But is it True?: A Citizen's Guide to Environmental Health and Safety (Cambridge, MA: Harvard University Press, 1995).

Wilkinson, Chris F. "Being More Realistic About Chemical Carcinogenesis." www.pmep.cce.cornell.edu/facts-slides-self-facts/gen-pubre-carcin-wilkinson.

Willet, W.C. "Balancing life-style and genomics research for disease prevention," Science, 2002, v.296: 695-698.

Wilson Schaef, Anne and Diane Faisel. The Addictive Organization: Why We Overwork, Cover Up, Pick Up th Pieces, Please the Boss and Perpetuate Sick Organizations (NY: HarperOne, 1990).

Winston, Mark L. Nature Wars: People vs. Pests (Cambridge, MA: Harvard University Press, 1997).

Wisconsin Ag Connection. "Hebl Decides to Drop Legislation to Ban Atrazine in Wisconsin," (February 18, 2010). www.wisconsinagconnection.com/Story-State.php?Id=202.

Witt, (HBO Studios, DVD, 2004).

World Conference on Breast Cancer Foundation. www.wcbcf.ca/foundation/profile.

World Population Review. www.worldpopulationreview.com/us-cities/lincoln-population.

Ziem, Grace. "Understanding Patients with Multiple Chemical Sensitivity," Letters to the Editor, American Family Physician. www.aafp.org/afp/990415ap/letters.

REVIEWS

Dr. Meriel Watts, Pesticide Action Network, New Zealand:
"The title says it all: 'avoidable human suffering.' That's pesticides. It is unconscionable that powerful interests obfuscate and deny, and innocent people continue to be unknowingly exposed to chemicals that will take their lives, leaving others to grieve and pick up the pieces, all in the name of profit for the few. This book is a story of love and loss, of hope and hopelessness and the pesticides that blight so many young lives. A must read for anyone who thinks all is well in the collided worlds of farming, chemicals and politics."
****

Dr. Werner Muller, Professor Emeritus of Science Education, New Mexico Highlands University; Rancher, Las Vegas, San Miguel County, New Mexico:
"Every chemistry major, in addition to those in the environmental sciences, should read this book, to know that as they become enamored with their ability to synthesize new compounds, they do extraordinary things to people, and realize they are dabbling in a discipline that carries enormous moral and ethical responsibility for the health of the human race and the environment."
****

Dr. Dan Bishop, Professor Emeritus of Chemistry, Colorado State University:
"There is a need for this book. The American Conscience must somehow be awakened from its drug-induced lethargy. As this book points out so clearly, 'collateral damage' and 'acceptable risk' are terms that have no moral currency when the outcome is measured in the avoidable loss of human lives. The use of real-life human-interest stories ... draw the reader into the topic reminding the reader that behind those numbers and statistics are real human beings whose lives are at stake."
****

Author's Bio

Ron Wooten-Green, Ph.D., author of <u>When the Dying Speak: How to Listen to and Learn from Those Facing Death</u>, is a Political Scientist specializing in Research Methodology and, as a hospice chaplain, has ministered to approximately 1000 hospice patients and families in Iowa and Nebraska. Raised on a dairy farm in Central NY, he served as Assistant 4-H Agent as a young man, and now lives with his wife, Linda, in Cuenca, Ecuador. He can be reached at <u>wootengreen@msn.com</u>.

www.ingramcontent.com/pod-product-compliance
Lightning Source LLC
Chambersburg PA
CBHW072302200526
45168CB00014B/154